SBAs, EMQs & SAQs in
PRACTICE PAPERS

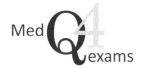

Matthew Hanks

tfm Publishing Limited, Castle Hill Barns, Harley, Shrewsbury, SY5 6LX, UK
Tel: +44 (0)1952 510061; Fax: +44 (0)1952 510192
E-mail: info@tfmpublishing.com; Web site: www.tfmpublishing.com

Editing, design & typesetting: Nikki Bramhill BSc Hons Dip Law
Cover photo: © iStock.com
Female doctor or surgeon with stethoscope in the hands (Igor Vershinsky) — stock
photo ID: 1221847703

First edition:	© 2021
Paperback	ISBN: 978-1-913755-04-1
E-book editions:	© 2021
ePub	ISBN: 978-1-913755-05-8
Mobi	ISBN: 978-1-913755-06-5
Web pdf	ISBN: 978-1-913755-07-2

Printed by Gutenberg Press Ltd., Gudja Road, Tarxien, GXQ 2902, Malta
Tel: +356 2398 2201; Fax: +356 2398 2290
E-mail: info@gutenberg.com.mt; Web site: www.gutenberg.com.mt

Contents

About the Editor

Dr. Matthew Hanks graduated from the University of Sheffield in 2015 with an MBChB in medicine; prior to this Matthew studied for a BSc Biomedical Science degree in Sheffield graduating in 2010 with a first class honours degree. He has a keen interest in teaching and has devised many different teaching programmes for students which have been engaging and received positive feedback. He now hopes to take this passion further by providing students with resources that are both useful and informative to enhance their learning opportunities.

Contributors

Dr. Gemma Adams MBChB
Clinical Fellow in General Medicine and Geriatrics, South Yorkshire Deanery

Dr. Jack Baskerville BMedSci MBChB
Locum Senior House Officer, South Yorkshire Region

Dr. Paul Galaway BA MBBS MRCP
CT2 Core Medical Trainee, South Yorkshire Deanery

Miss Rose Gnap BSc (Hons) BMBS PGCert MRCSEd
CT2 Core Surgical Trainee, East Midlands North Deanery

Dr. Richard Harold MBChB (Hons)
Locum Senior House Officer, South Yorkshire Region

Dr. Mei-Ling Henry BMedSci BMBS
CT2 Core Surgical Trainee, East Midlands North Deanery

Dr. Amelia Lloyd BMedSci MBChB
F2 Sandwell and West Birmingham Hospitals NHS Trust

Dr. Rebecca Marlor BMedSci (Hons) MBChB
CT2 Core Medical Trainee, South Yorkshire Deanery

Dr. Katherine McPhail BMedSci MBChB
Clinical Fellow in Critical Care, Northern Deanery

Dr. Morwenna Read BMedSci (Hons) MBChB (Hons)
F2 Sheffield Teaching Hospitals NHS Foundation Trust

Dr. Emily Reed BMedSci MBChB
F2 Sheffield Teaching Hospitals NHS Foundation Trust

Dr. Chloe Theodorou BMBS
CT1 Core Surgical Trainee, North Western Deanery

Dr. Emma Whitehall BMedSci MBChB (Hons)
CT2 Core Surgical Trainee, East Midlands North Deanery

Acknowledgements

I would like to thank all those who have taken the time to contribute to this title which is the amalgamation of knowledge from professionals studying and working all over the United Kingdom; without their hard work and dedication, this book would not have been possible.

I would like to thank Megan Ward and Glenda Hanks for their patience whilst the book has taken shape and the many nights of proofreading the text to ensure it will be useful for students. Koda and Joel Ward have provided a useful distraction when required!

Mrs Maxine Ward and Mrs Lisa Wheatley have been instrumental in locating many of the ECGs in this book and without their hard work and dedication the high-quality images in this publication would not have been possible.

Finally, the road to medical finals is a long one and this is the last major hurdle to becoming a doctor; the many hours of hard work and dedication already demonstrated in getting this far is about to pay off. All that is left to say is good luck!

Matthew Hanks
May 2021

Normal reference values

Please note normal reference values may vary between different hospitals.

Hb	Male 131-166g/L
	Female 110-147g/L
MCV	81-96fL
Platelets	150-400 x 10^9/L
WCC	3.5-9.5 x 10^9/L
Neutrophils	1.7-6.5 x 10^9/L
Lymphocytes	1.0-3.0 x 10^9/L
Eosinophils	0.04-0.5 x 10^9/L
Basophils	0.0-0.25 x 10^9/L
Sodium	133-146mmol/L
Potassium	3.5-5.3mmol/L
Urea	2.5-7.8mmol/L
Creatinine	62-106µmol/L
eGFR	>90
Calcium	2.25-2.5mmol/L
Total protein	60-80g/L
Globulin	18-36g/L
Bilirubin	0-21µmol/L
ALT	0-41iU/L
ALP	30-130iU/L

AST	0-35iU/L
Albumin	35-50g/L

PT	10.1-11.8 seconds
APTT	20.2-28.7 seconds
Thrombin time	11.3-17.4 seconds
Fibrinogen	2.0-4.0g/L

CRP	0-5mg/L

Abbreviations

Ab	Antibody
ABG	Arterial blood gas
ABPI	Ankle Brachial Pressure Index
ACE	Angiotensin-converting enzyme
ACTH	Adrenocorticotrophic hormone
ADP	Adenosine diphosphate
AF	Atrial fibrillation
AKI	Acute kidney injury
ALP	Alkaline phosphatase
ALT	Alanine aminotransferase
ANA	Antinuclear antibody
ANCA	Anti-neutrophil cytoplasmic antibody
Anti-GAD	Anti-glutamic acid decarboxylase
Anti-GBM	Anti-glomerular basement membrane
APTT	Activated partial thromboplastin time
ARDS	Acute respiratory distress syndrome
ARMD	Age-related macular degeneration
ASD	Atrial septal defect
AST	Aspartate aminotransferase
ATP	Adenosine triphosphate
BCG	Bacille Calmette-Guérin
BP	Blood pressure
bpm	Beats per minute
CA-19	Cancer antigen
CEA	Carcinoembryonic antigen
CJD	Creutzfeldt-Jakob disease
CKD	Chronic kidney disease

Cl⁻	Chloride
CNS	Central nervous system
COPD	Chronic obstructive pulmonary disease
COX	Cyclo-oxygenase
CREST	Calcinosis, Raynaud's phenomenon, oesophageal dysmotility, sclerodactyly and telangiectasia
CRP	C-reactive protein
CSF	Cerebrospinal fluid
CT	Computed tomography
CVD	Cardiovascular disease
DIC	Disseminated intravascular coagulation
DKA	Diabetic ketoacidosis
DOAC	Direct oral anticoagulant
DTaP	Diphtheria, tetanus and pertussis
ECG	Electrocardiogram
ENT	Ear, nose and throat
ERCP	Endoscopic retrograde cholangiopancreatography
ESR	Erythrocyte sedimentation rate
FAP	Familial adenomatous polyposis
FBC	Full blood count
GCS	Glasgow Coma Scale
GFR	Glomerular filtration rate
GORD	Gastro-oesophageal reflux disease
GTN	Glyceryl trinitrate
H⁺	Hydrogen
Hb	Haemoglobin
HCO₃⁻	Bicarbonates
Hep B	Hepatitis B
HiB	Haemophilus influenzae B
HIV	Human immunodeficiency virus
HMG-CoA	3-hydroxy-3-methylglutaryl coenzyme A
HNPCC	Hereditary non-polyposis colorectal cancer
HPV	Human papilloma virus

HR	Heart rate
HUS	Haemolytic uraemic syndrome
INR	International Normalised Ratio
IPV	Inactivated polio vaccine
IV	Intravenous
IVDU	Intravenous drug user
JVP	Jugular venous pressure
K⁺	Potassium
LFT	Liver function test
LLETZ	Large loop excision of the transformation zone
LUTS	Lower urinary tract symptoms
MAHA	Microangiopathic haemolytic anaemia
MALT	Mucosa-associated lymphoid tissue
MAP	MYH-associated polyposis
MCV	Mean corpuscular volume
MDT	Multidisciplinary team
MEN	Multiple endocrine neoplasia
MenACWY	Meningitis A, C, W, Y
Men B	Meningitis B
MI	Myocardial infarction
MMR	Measles, mumps and rubella
MRI	Magnetic resonance imaging
Na⁺	Sodium
NSAID	Non-steroidal anti-inflammatory drug
NSTEMI	Non-ST elevation myocardial infarction
OGD	Oesophageal gastroduodenoscopy
PaCO₂	Partial pressure of carbon dioxide
PAN	Polyarteritis nodosa
PaO₂	Partial pressure of oxygen
PCT	Proximal convoluted tubule
PCV	Pneumococcal conjugate vaccine
PET	Positron emission tomography
PPI	Proton pump inhibitor

PPV	Positive predictive value
PSA	Prostate-specific antigen
PT	Prothrombin time
PVD	Peripheral vascular disease
REM	Rapid eye movement
RR	Respiratory rate
RTC	Road traffic collision
STEMI	ST-elevation myocardial infarction
STI	Sexually transmitted infection
T3	Tri-iodothyronine
T4	Thyroxine
TACO	Transfusion-associated circulatory overload
Td	Tetanus and diphtheria
TNM	Tumour, node, metastasis
TPO	Thyroid peroxidase antibodies
TRALI	Transfusion-related acute lung injury
TSH	Thyroid-stimulating hormone
TTP	Thrombotic thrombocytopenic purpura
TURP	Transurethral resection of the prostate
U&E	Urea & Electrolytes
UTI	Urinary tract infection
VSD	Ventriculoseptal defect
WCC	White cell count

Section 1

Questions

Chapter 1

Practice paper 1
QUESTIONS

Single best answer questions

1) A 38-year-old male presents to the emergency department with an 8-hour history of retrosternal chest pain which radiates to the right arm. The pain is worst on inspiration and is eased by leaning forward. On examination, a pericardial friction rub is heard which is heard best on expiration and is loudest at the left sternal edge. What is the most appropriate diagnosis?

a.   Myocardial infarction.
b.   Pericarditis.
c.   Angina.
d.   Costochondritis.

2) A 54-year-old female with known COPD develops a pneumothorax. On chest X-ray, the pneumothorax is measured as 1cm. She is not breathless. What is the most appropriate initial management?

a.   Aspiration.
b.   Chest drain.
c.   No treatment.
d.   High-flow oxygen.

3) A 34-year-old male presents to his primary care doctor with a 2-month history of dyspepsia and intermittent epigastric pain that occurs after food. He has noticed recently that he has a dry cough in the morning. He denies any weight loss, dysphagia or vomiting. He undergoes an oesophageal gastroduodenoscopy (OGD) which shows a 4cm segment of oesophagus which appears abnormal; biopsies show metaplasia from stratified squamous cells to simple columnar cells. What is the most likely diagnosis?

a. Peptic ulcer disease.
b. Hiatus hernia.
c. Barrett's oesophagus.
d. Tropical sprue.

4) A patient presents to the emergency department hypotensive, feverish and with a difficulty in breathing. They give a history of a productive cough of green sputum for 3 days. Blood results show a CRP of 154mg/L and a new acute kidney injury. A chest X-ray shows evidence of a right basal pneumonia. What is the mechanism behind their kidney injury?

a. Pre-renal: hypoperfusion of the kidneys secondary to hypovolaemia and systemic vasodilation.
b. Intrinsic: acute tubular necrosis secondary to nephrotoxins.
c. Post-renal: urinary outflow obstruction.
d. Glomerulonephritis: immune complex deposition in mesangial cells.

5) Which of the following anti-diabetic medications would not cause hypoglycaemia?

a. Gliclazide.
b. Metformin.
c. Humalog Mix 50.
d. NovoRapid®.

6) A 29-year-old male with generalised tonic clonic seizures develops a fever and flu-like symptoms. A few days later, his skin began to turn red before blistering and peeling. He also has painful crusts and erosions in his mouth. Two weeks prior, his antiepileptic medication had been changed. Which antiepileptic drug is the most likely cause of his symptoms?

a. Ethosuximide.
b. Levetiracetam.
c. Lamotrigine.
d. Topiramate.

7) Which of the following patients would be appropriate for blood transfusion according to current guidance?

a. A 67-year-old male with CKD 4 with a Hb of 86g/dL.
b. A 75-year-old male with previous ischaemic heart disease, attends his primary care doctor due to an increasing frequency of angina attacks. His Hb is 76g/dL.
c. An asymptomatic 45-year-old female with a Hb of 78g/dL.
d. A 72-year-old female who is tired, with a Hb of 101g/dL.

8) A 28-year-old male presents to the emergency department following a dog bite. He is normally fit and well, has no allergies and takes no regular medications. He has sustained two bites, one on his left forearm and the other on his left hand. His wounds are cleaned and dressed, and he is given a tetanus booster; due to the location of the wound he is at a high risk of a wound infection. What antibiotic would you prescribe for this patient?

a. Erythromycin.
b. Metronidazole.
c. Doxycycline.
d. Co-amoxiclav.

9) A 67-year-old female is diagnosed with dermatomyositis as part of a paraneoplastic syndrome. Which of the following cancers is least associated with dermatomyositis?

a. Breast cancer.
b. Lung cancer.
c. Malignant melanoma.
d. Gastric cancer.

10) A 45-year-old Asian male presents to the surgical outpatient clinic with a 4-month history of right upper quadrant pain, malaise and weight loss. He is known to have hepatitis B. On examination, a mass can be felt in the right upper quadrant with the presence of abdominal distention and shifting dullness. Bloods tests reveal a raised CRP and an elevated α-fetoprotein. What is the most likely diagnosis?

a. Cholangiocarcinoma.
b. Bacterial pneumonia.
c. Hepatocellular carcinoma.
d. Liver abscess.

11) Which of the following tumour markers is associated with colorectal cancer?

a. Alpha-fetoprotein.
b. Carcinoembryonic antigen.
c. Carcinoma antigen 125.
d. Carcinoma antigen 19-9.

12) Which of these medications does not list gynaecomastia as a side effect?

a. Digoxin.
b. Spironolactone.
c. Bisoprolol.
d. Amiodarone.

13) What is the most common presentation of a UTI in the elderly?

a. Delirium.
b. New-onset urinary incontinence.
c. Decreased mobility.
d. All of the above.

14) Which of the following would you not expect to see on a CT of the head of someone with hydrocephalus?

a. Ventricular dilatation.
b. Obstructing tumour.
c. Bony malformation.
d. Blood in bilateral ventricles.

15) A 21-year-old female presents to the emergency department with shortness of breath, fatigue, dizziness and pain on walking; the symptoms have progressively worsened and she feels her muscles are weaker in her upper limbs than 12 months ago. On examination, peripheral pulses are diminished and there is a difference between the systolic blood pressure readings in her arms and legs. Bloods reveal an ESR >40mm/h. What is the underlying diagnosis?

a.   Thoracic outlet syndrome.
b.   Subclavian steal syndrome.
c.   Giant cell arteritis.
d.   Takayasu's arteritis.

16) Which of the following is not an example of a fragility fracture?

a.   Base of fifth metatarsal fracture.
b.   Colles' distal radius fracture.
c.   Surgical neck of humerus fracture.
d.   Pubic ramus fracture.

17) Which electrolyte imbalance is difficult to manage unless magnesium is corrected first?

a.   Phosphate.
b.   Calcium.
c.   Sodium.
d.   Potassium.

18) What is the pathophysiology of Ménière's disease?

a. Increased endolymphatic pressure in the inner ear.
b. Otoliths in the semi-circular canal.
c. Reduced endolymphatic pressure in the inner ear.
d. Tearing of the vestibulocochlear nerve.

19) An elderly female presents with a suspicious unilateral thyroid lump. She is told she has the most aggressive form of thyroid cancer with a very poor prognosis. What is likely to have been seen on biopsy?

a. Papillary carcinoma.
b. Anaplastic carcinoma.
c. Follicular carcinoma.
d. Medullary carcinoma.

20) A 65-year-old male with known atrial fibrillation attends the emergency department with a sudden loss of vision in his right eye. When he is reviewed, all symptoms have resolved. He describes the event as if a curtain was falling across his right eye. Fundoscopy is normal. What is the most likely diagnosis?

a. Multiple sclerosis.
b. Optic neuritis.
c. Amaurosis fugax.
d. Central retinal vein occlusion.

21) A 24-year-old male presents to the emergency department with a 4-day history of auditory hallucinations, paranoid delusions and psychomotor agitation. He has no past psychiatric history and has returned from a 1-week holiday where he used large amounts of cannabis and cocaine. What is the likely diagnosis?

a.   Acute intoxication.
b.   Delirium tremens.
c.   Drug-induced psychosis.
d.   Schizophrenia.

22) A 9-year-old boy presents with a widespread palpable purpuric rash on the backs of his legs and buttocks. A diagnosis of Henoch-Schönlein purpura is suspected. Which organ is not characteristically also affected in this condition?

a.   Joints.
b.   Gut.
c.   Kidneys.
d.   Lungs.

23) What is the ideal orientation of the fetal head to advance through the pelvis?

a.   Occipito-posterior.
b.   Occipito-transverse.
c.   Occipito-anterior.
d.   Brow.

24) Which of the following bacteria is most strongly associated with lesion production in acne vulgaris?

a. *Staphylococcus aureus.*
b. *Propionibacterium acnes.*
c. *Staphylococcus epidermidis.*
d. *Streptococcus viridans.*

25) A 78-year-old female attends pre-operative assessment prior to undergoing elective coronary artery bypass grafts. She has a past medical history of hypertension, angina and hypercholesterolaemia but is otherwise well. She is apyrexial and her examination is unremarkable. Blood results and chest X-ray are unremarkable; her urine dip is negative for leucocytes and nitrites. Routine groin swabs come back as positive for methicillin-resistant *Staphylococcus aureus*. What is the most appropriate initial management for this result?

a. Conservative management.
b. Topical decolonisation.
c. Oral flucloxacillin.
d. IV vancomycin.

26) A 52-year-old male presents to the emergency department with increasing shortness of breath 4 days after commencing a new medication to control his blood pressure. On examination, he has a stony dullness to both lung bases and chest X-ray reveals pulmonary oedema. What is the most likely cause?

a. Amiloride.
b. Amlodipine.
c. Hydralazine.
d. Ramipril.

27) Which of the following insulins may be used as a basal (background) insulin in the treatment of diabetes mellitus?

a.   NovoRapid®.
b.   Insulin degludec.
c.   Insulin aspart.
d.   Insulin lispro.

28) A 76-year-old female attends her primary care doctor with increased ankle swelling and shortness of breath. The primary care doctor is concerned about heart failure and prescribes furosemide. What is the mechanism of action of this drug?

a.   Inhibits bicarbonate reabsorption at the proximal tubule.
b.   Inhibits Na^+/Cl^- in the early distal tubule.
c.   Inhibits $Na^+/K^+/Cl^-$ in the thick ascending limb.
d.   Inhibits Na^+ and water reabsorption in the collecting duct.

29) A 65-year-old male attends the urology clinic with a 4-week history of haematuria. He undergoes a cystoscopy which shows a large mass in the bladder. What is the most common form of bladder cancer?

a.   Transitional cell carcinoma.
b.   Squamous cell carcinoma.
c.   Adenocarcinoma.
d.   Sarcoma.

30) A 72-year-old female with known atrial fibrillation presents to the emergency department with weakness in her right arm and face; her husband noticed her face drooping 30 minutes ago. She does not currently take any medication. The doctor diagnoses a stroke. What type of stroke is likely to have occurred?

a. Embolic.
b. Haemorrhagic.
c. Thrombosis.
d. Hypoperfusion.

31) As part of routine monitoring, a 30-year-old patient with HIV undergoes an ECG. The patient is currently well with no other health problems. They do not have any chest pain or shortness of breath. What is the most likely diagnosis?

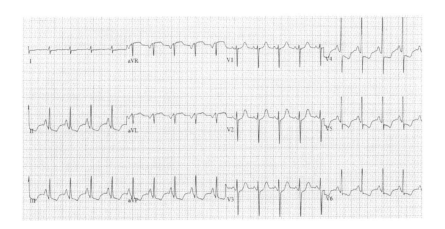

a. Inferior NSTEMI.
b. Myocarditis.
c. Pericarditis.
d. Posterior STEMI.

32) A 75-year-old female is admitted to the emergency department following a collapse at home; she initially felt dizzy and lost her balance prior to falling. She did not hit her head or injure herself. An ECG is performed to assess for an underlying cause for the collapse. What does the ECG show?

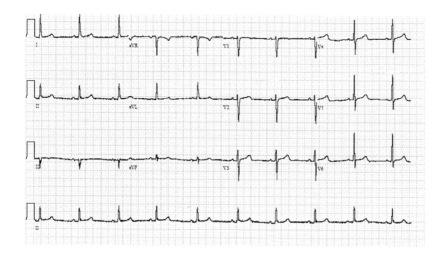

a. Normal sinus rhythm.
b. Sinus tachycardia.
c. Sinus bradycardia.
d. Complete heart block.

33) A 65-year-old male presents to the emergency department with a gradual onset of shortness of breath. What is the most likely diagnosis from the chest X-ray below?

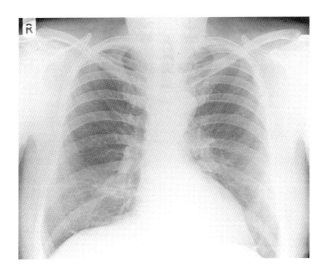

a.   Chronic obstructive pulmonary disease.
b.   Right lower lobe lesion.
c.   Right middle lobe lesion.
d.   Pulmonary tuberculosis.

34) A 28-year-old male is reviewed by his primary care doctor with a 2-month history of shortness of breath. A chest radiograph is taken to investigate these symptoms further. What does this image show?

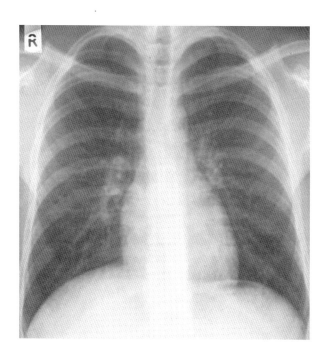

a.   Normal chest X-ray.
b.   Right pneumothorax.
c.   Left pneumothorax.
d.   Right pleural effusion.

35) You are a junior doctor on a respiratory ward round and review a patient with the consultant who hands you the latest ABG result and asks you to interpret the readings. The patient is not currently on oxygen. What does the ABG show?

	Result	Normal values
pH	7.36	7.35-7.45
$PaCO_2$	4.1	4.7-6.0kPa
HCO_3^-	21	24-30mmol/L
PaO_2	13	11-13 on room air
Base excess	-6	+/- 2mmol/L
Anion gap	14	12-16 mmol/L

a.   Compensated metabolic acidosis.
b.   Uncompensated metabolic acidosis.
c.   Compensated respiratory acidosis.
d.   Uncompensated respiratory acidosis.

36) You are the doctor on-call and have been asked to review a 48-year-old female who is 12 hours post-laparoscopic cholecystectomy She has been given regular opioid medication since the procedure for pain control. The nursing staff are concerned about her reduced level of consciousness, reduced respiratory rate and constricted pupils. An ABG is performed on 15L of oxygen on a non-rebreathe mask. What does the ABG show?

	Result	Normal values
pH	7.26	7.35-7.45
$PaCO_2$	7.1	4.7-6.0kPa
HCO_3^-	28	24-30mmol/L
PaO_2	12	11-13 on room air
Base excess	+2	+/- 2mmol/L
Anion gap	14	12-16mmol/L

a.   Compensated metabolic acidosis.
b.   Uncompensated metabolic acidosis.
c.   Compensated respiratory acidosis.
d.   Uncompensated respiratory acidosis.

37) A 62-year-old female with known COPD is admitted with shortness of breath and a fever. She is placed on a 40% venturi mask. What does the ABG show?

	Result	Normal values
pH	7.43	7.35-7.45
$PaCO_2$	6.5	4.7-6.0kPa
HCO_3^-	19	24-30mmol/L
PaO_2	15	11-13 on room air
Base excess	+1	+/- 2mmol/L
Anion gap	14	12-16mmol/L

a.   Compensated metabolic alkalosis.
b.   Uncompensated metabolic alkalosis.
c.   Compensated respiratory alkalosis.
d.   Uncompensated respiratory alkalosis.

38) A 45-year-old female presents to the emergency department following a flight to New York with her partner. She returned 24 hours ago and has been experiencing shortness of breath for the past 16 hours. On examination, she has a right swollen calf. She is commenced on 4L of oxygen by a nasal cannula and an ABG is taken to assess for respiratory pathology. What does the ABG show?

	Result	Normal values
pH	7.49	7.35-7.45
PaCO$_2$	4.8	4.7-6.0kPa
HCO$_3^-$	25	24-30mmol/L
PaO$_2$	9	11-13 on room air
Base excess	-2	+/- 2mmol/L
Anion gap	13	12-16mmol/L

a.   Compensated metabolic alkalosis.
b.   Uncompensated metabolic alkalosis.
c.   Compensated respiratory alkalosis.
d.   Uncompensated respiratory alkalosis.

39) A 45-year-old female presents to the emergency department following a flight to New York with her partner. She returned 24 hours ago and has been experiencing shortness of breath for the past 16 hours. On examination, she has a right swollen calf. She is commenced on 4L of oxygen by a nasal cannula and an ABG is taken to assess for respiratory pathology. What does the ABG show?

	Result	Normal values
pH	7.49	7.35-7.45
PaCO$_2$	4.8	4.7-6.0kPa
HCO$_3^-$	25	24-30mmol/L
PaO$_2$	9	11-13 on room air
Base excess	-2	+/- 2mmol/L
Anion gap	13	12-16mmol/L

a.   Type I respiratory failure.
b.   Type II respiratory failure.
c.   Compensated respiratory alkalosis.
d.   Uncompensated respiratory acidosis.

40) A 28-year-old male was admitted with persistent vomiting for the past 48 hours. An ABG was taken to assess the severity of his condition on room air. What does the ABG show?

	Result	Normal values
pH	7.56	7.35-7.45
$PaCO_2$	5.0	4.7-6.0kPa
HCO_3^-	30	24-30mmol/L
PaO_2	13	11-13 on room air
Base excess	+6	+/- 2mmol/L
Anion gap	13	12-16mmol/L

a. Compensated metabolic alkalosis
b. Uncompensated metabolic alkalosis
c. Compensated respiratory alkalosis
d. Uncompensated respiratory alkalosis

Chapter 2

Practice paper 2
QUESTIONS

Extended matching questions

Structural heart syndromes

a. Tetralogy of Fallot.
b. Williams syndrome.
c. Bicuspid aortic valve.
d. Ventricular septal defect.

e. Atrial septal defect.
f. Coarctation of the aorta.
g. Dextrocardia.
h. Pulmonary atresia.

Match the description of the patient with the most likely diagnosis.

1) A patient is found to have supravalvular stenosis on echocardiography. They have a background history of anxiety, mild learning difficulties, unusual facies and a small habitus.

2) A 20-year-old develops shortness of breath and angina on exertion. On examination, there is an ejection systolic murmur.

3) A 1-year-old child is found to have a harsh systolic murmur, loudest at the left sternal edge, and left sternal heave.

4) A 5-year-old with recurrent chest infections is found to have very small QRS complexes in the lateral leads of his ECG.

5) A 30-year-old patient develops dense left-sided paresis following a coughing fit.

Pleural effusions

a.	Congestive cardiac failure.	e.	Malignancy.
b.	Hypothyroidism.	f.	Renal failure.
c.	Liver failure.	g.	Rheumatoid arthritis.
d.	Meigs syndrome.	h.	Tuberculosis.

Match the description of the patient with the most likely diagnosis.

6) A patient presents with worsening shortness of breath. There is marked ascites, bruising and jaundice noted. There are bilateral pleural effusions.

7) A patient presents with a 2-month history of weight loss and night sweats. There is inguinal and cervical lymphadenopathy. There is a unilateral pleural effusion.

8) A patient presents with a 6-month history of weight loss and night sweats. The patient is an ex-IVDU and has been homeless until recently. There is bilateral cervical lymphadenopathy and it is possible to percuss a right-sided pleural effusion.

9) A patient presents with worsening shortness of breath and oliguria. There is marked ascites. There are bilateral pleural effusions.

10) A patient presents with a history of fatigue and weight gain. There is mild peripheral oedema, dry skin and they appear pale. A chest radiograph identifies bilateral pleural effusions.

Gastrointestinal infections

a. *Staphylococcus aureus.*	e. *Clostridium difficile.*
b. *Campylobacter.*	f. *Bacillus cereus.*
c. *Escherichia coli.*	g. Rotavirus.
d. *Vibrio cholerae.*	h. Norovirus.

Match the description of the patient with the most likely underlying cause for their infection.

11) An 18-year-old student orders a Chinese takeaway and is unable to finish the complete meal. The next day he reheats the rice and noodles and experiences profuse diarrhoea and vomiting.

12) A 42-year-old male is admitted to the emergency department following a circumcision 2 weeks ago; the operative site is red and warm. He is treated for a postoperative wound infection and given a course of oral antibiotics. He experiences abdominal pain and profuse bloody diarrhoea 48 hours after commencing antibiotics. The medical staff were unaware he had two courses of antibiotics as an inpatient following his surgical procedure.

13) A 20-year-old female has diarrhoea and vomiting 4 hours after eating at a new restaurant in her local city; her partner who also ate the same meal is experiencing these symptoms. The condition resolves with 24 hours.

14) A 20-year-old male is travelling on his gap year around India and experiences profuse diarrhoea. He attends the local hospital with profound dehydration. The doctor describes his stools as rice water.

15) A 30-year-old hospital porter is admitted with nausea, vomiting, headache and watery diarrhoea. He has experienced weakness and headaches. He notes he transported a patient with diarrhoea 24 hours prior to commencement of symptoms.

Haematuria

a.   Renal calculi.

b.   Nephritic syndrome.

c.   Catheter-related trauma.

d.   Renal cell carcinoma.

e.   IgA nephropathy.

f.   Penile trauma.

g.   Anti-GBM disease.

h.   Bladder cancer.

Match the description of the patient with the most likely diagnosis.

16) A 46-year-old male smoker presents with a 6-week history of intermittent haematuria, weight loss and left flank pain.

17) A 92-year-old male with a long-term urethral catheter presents with a blood-stained catheter bag. He has severe dementia and appears distressed, grabbing at his clothes pulling his cannula out.

18) A 65-year-old patient presents with generalised symptoms of weight loss, fatigue and cachexia. A chest X-ray shows multiple small lesions on the bases of the lungs and urine dipstick reveals haematuria.

19) Often presents with hypertension, oliguria and proteinuria. Haematuria often is microscopic.

20) Patients suffering with this condition may present with severe haematuria, with clots, requiring '3-way' catheterisation.

Endocrine investigations

a. Anti-GAD and islet cell antibodies.
b. Dexamethasone suppression test.
c. TSH receptor antibodies.
d. Anti-thyroid peroxidase antibodies.
e. Serum ACE level.
f. HbA1c.
g. Serum aldosterone level.
h. Glucose tolerance test.

Match the below presentations with the most appropriate investigation.

21) A 25-year-old male presents to his primary care doctor complaining of polyuria and polydipsia; he has no past medical history of note. The primary care doctor is concerned about Type 1 diabetes and orders relevant investigations.

22) A 40-year-old presents to his primary care doctor with anxiety, increased sweating, palpitations and weight loss. On examination, he has a fine tremor and warm moist skin. The primary care doctor would like to investigate for Graves' disease.

23) A 50-year-old female presents to her primary care doctor with dry skin, hoarseness of voice and constipation. She also has a neck swelling which is new and the primary care doctor would like to investigate for Hashimoto's disease.

24) A patient presents to their primary care doctor with weight gain and fatigue. They have noticed they have put on a lot of weight around their abdomen and also think their skin is much thinner and have what look like stretch marks developing — purple marks on their abdomen, which are tender to touch. The primary care doctor would like to arrange investigations for Cushing's syndrome.

25) A 55-year-old male presents to his primary care doctor as his hat and shoes no longer appear to fit. As well as this his wedding ring is much tighter than previously and he has severely painful joints. The primary care doctor would like to investigate for acromegaly.

Confusion

a. Alzheimer's disease.
b. Creutzfeldt-Jacob disease.
c. Dementia with Lewy bodies.
d. Normal pressure hydrocephalus.
e. Vascular dementia.
f. Korsakoff's syndrome.
g. Frontotemporal dementia.
h. Depression.

Match the description of the patient with the most likely diagnosis.

26) An 82-year-old male with a past medical history of ischaemic heart disease, hypertension and diabetes presents with memory problems. His family report that these started quite suddenly last year and got noticeably worse abruptly a few months later.

27) A 77-year-old male presents with memory problems. He has also been experiencing recurrent hallucinations of people in his house, which have been distressing him greatly. According to his family, his confusion fluctuates considerably from day to day.

28) A 72-year-old female presents with a personality change. Her family report that she has become apathetic and does not pay attention to them. She lives alone and they are concerned because she has stopped doing housework and has been eating large amounts of unhealthy food. She often answers the door to them in her underwear, something very out of character for her.

29) An 83-year-old female presents with memory problems and mobility issues. She finds that she is very forgetful and that it takes her a long time to process thoughts. She thinks that the problems have been going on for several months; however, her son thinks that her walking has looked strange for some time longer than this and reports she has lost continence of urine. On examination, she walks slowly, with a broad-based, shuffling gait. Tone is normal.

30) An 85-year-old male with a history of diabetes and hypercholesterolaemia presents with memory impairment. He and his family have noticed a gradual deterioration in his memory over several months, with him often forgetting names of family members and recent conversations and events.

Haemoglobin

a. Hb A.
b. Hb S.
c. Hb F.
d. Hb C.

e. Alpha thalassaemia minor.
f. Beta thalassaemia major.
g. High affinity for oxygen.
h. Low affinity for oxygen.

Match the type of haemoglobin with the description below.

31) Composed of two alpha and two beta chains.

32) As a result of the deletion of 1-4 of the alpha-globulin genes coding haemoglobin molecules.

33) Results in recurrent painful crises and chronic haemolytic anaemia.

34) Consists of two alpha and two gamma subunits.

35) Adult haemoglobin has a _____ compared with fetal haemoglobin.

Parasites

a. Schistosomiasis.
b. African trypanosomiasis.
c. Cutaneous leishmaniasis.
d. Cutaneous larva migrans.

e. Loa loa.
f. Visceral leishmaniasis.
g. Amoebiasis.
h. Lymphatic filariasis.

Match the description to the most suitable organism.

36) A 24-year-old female has recently returned from a holiday in the Caribbean; during this time she spent a lot of time on the beach and has developed an intensely itchy rash. On examination, there are snake-like tracks on her foot.

37) A 34-year-old male presents to his primary care doctor with a nodule on his ankle. On examination, it has ulcerated. He reports that this is at the site of an insect bite he sustained several months ago in South Africa.

38) An 18-year-old presents with painless haematuria and increased urinary frequency after returning from his gap year. He finished his trip in Africa and swam in Lake Malawi just prior to coming home.

39) Transmitted by the tsetse fly, patients can end up in a coma.

40) A 36-year-old female presents with pain in her right eye. On examination, a worm is seen crossing the conjunctiva. Blood results show an increased eosinophil count and a raised level of IgE.

Neurological consequences of rheumatological disease

a.	Visual field defect.	e.	Atlanto-axial subluxation.
b.	Brachial plexopathy.	f.	Oculomotor nerve palsy.
c.	Carpal tunnel syndrome.	g.	Meningoencephalitis.
d.	Mononeuritis multiplex.	h.	Psychosis.

Match the description of the patient with the most likely diagnosis.

41) A 67-year-old female with rheumatoid arthritis complains of longstanding neck pain. She is finding it increasingly difficult to walk due to clumsiness and lack of coordination. Plantar reflexes are upgoing on examination.

42) An 80-year-old male newly diagnosed with giant cell arteritis presents with double vision when looking straight ahead. On examination, his right eye looks downwards and laterally.

43) A male with polyarteritis nodosum complains of right-sided weakness of wrist extension. He mentions longstanding loss of sensation of the dorsum of his right foot and anterior shin.

44) A female with rheumatoid arthritis complains of pain and tingling in her thumb, index and middle fingers.

45) An 85-year-old male, who has just started treatment for giant cell arteritis, becomes withdrawn and irritable. He attempts to self-discharge from hospital as he claims the nursing staff are trying to kill him and has heard them talking about their plans to throw him out of the window.

Pancreaticobiliary malignancy

a.   Pancreatic adenocarcinoma.   e.   MEN Type 2A.
b.   Carcinoma of head of pancreas.   f.   MEN Type 2B.
c.   Primary biliary sclerosis.   g.   Cholangiocarcinoma.
d.   MEN Type 1.   h.   Gallbladder adenocarcinoma.

Match the description of the patient with the most likely diagnosis.

46)   A 32-year-old male attends the surgical outpatient clinic for review following diagnosis of a pancreatic tumour. Bloods show a primary hyperparathyroidism and a staging CT shows a concurrent pituitary adenoma.

47)   A 52-year-old male with a marfanoid habitus presents to his primary care doctor following a diagnosis of medullary thyroid carcinoma. He is concerned as further investigations have noted a phaeochromocytoma. He is worried that he may have other undiagnosed tumours.

48)   A 54-year-old female presents with a 6-month history of painless jaundice, weight loss and epigastric pain. She reports for the past 2 weeks she has had pale stools and dark urine. On examination, the gallbladder is palpable but non-tender.

49)   A 64-year-old male with known primary sclerosing cholangitis presents with a 4-week history of painless obstructive jaundice. He has noticed his clothes feel loose compared to last year and stools appear to float. On examination, hepatomegaly is evident but the gallbladder is not palpable.

50)   A 63-year-old male undergoes a laparoscopic cholecystectomy for acute cholecystitis. Following the removal of the gallbladder it is sent to the pathology lab and this incidental finding is made.

Postoperative complications

a. Abdominal ultrasound.
b. Abdominal X-ray.
c. Barium enema.
d. CT abdomen.
e. Full blood count.
f. Serum amylase.
g. Urinary amylase.
h. Wound swab.

Match the description of the patient with the most useful investigation.

51) A 32-year-old male has completed a course of high-dose steroids 1 week ago for Crohn's disease. He attends the emergency department with epigastric pain radiating to his back.

52) A 58-year-old female presents with left iliac fossa pain. On examination, she is pyrexial and tachycardic, and has localised tenderness in the left iliac fossa.

53) A 19-year-old female presents with right iliac fossa pain. On examination, she has localised tenderness in the right iliac fossa, but her observations are normal.

54) A 71-year-old male has had a Hartmann's procedure 3 days ago for a sigmoid colon tumour. The junior doctor is called to see him because he is vomiting and has not opened his bowels since surgery. On examination, his abdomen is distended and generally tender.

55) A 31-year-old obese male has had an open inguinal hernia repair 4 days previously. He visits his primary care doctor because he feels generally unwell. On examination, he is pyrexial and there is purulent fluid seeping through his dressing.

Breast pathology

a. Fibroadenoma.   e. Lipoma.
b. Fat necrosis.   f. Seroma.
c. Lobular carcinoma.   g. Phyllodes tumour.
d. Ductal carcinoma *in situ*.   h. Breast cyst.

Match the description of the patient with the most likely diagnosis.

56) A 22-year-old female presents to the breast clinic with a 5-day history of a small lump in the upper outer quadrant of her left breast. She is concerned as her mother, grandmother and aunt have had breast cancer. She denies any history of trauma or pregnancy. On examination, the lump is smooth, mobile and 1cm in size.

57) A 30-year-old female is seen in clinic 10 days after undergoing a right mastectomy and axillary node clearance. She has noticed a swelling in the same breast that has slowly increased in size. It was initially non-tender but is now becoming increasingly painful. On examination, the lump appears to be soft and fluctuant.

58) A 34-year-old female presents to you with a 3-week history of right-sided breast pain. On examination, she is tender on palpation of the chest and there is some chest swelling.

59) A 52-year-old female undergoes breast screening and is noted to have microcalcifications on mammography. She has no symptoms and breast examination is normal.

60) A 45-year-old female comes to see you a month after a road traffic accident where she was the driver. Since then she has developed a lump over her right upper breast. When you examine it, this feels firm and seems to be made up of multiple small lumps.

Management of prostate disorders

a.	Alpha blocker.	e.	MRI of the prostate.
b.	5-alpha-reductase inhibitor.	f.	Transperineal prostate biopsy.
c.	TURP procedure.	g.	Radical prostatectomy.
d.	Transrectal ultrasound biopsy.	h.	Palliative radiotherapy.

Match the description with the most appropriate next step in management.

61) A 58-year-old male presents with LUTS which is evidenced in a bladder diary. His past medical history includes fainting episodes thought to be due to postural hypotension.

62) A 71-year-old male has had LUTS for several years successfully managed on pharmacological treatment. His primary care doctor has noticed an increasing PSA level over the last 12 months. His most recent reading is 6.5ng/ml.

63) A 67-year-old male has troublesome LUTS. He has been successfully managed on pharmacological treatment for many years but his symptoms have started to get worse over the last 6 months. His PSA level is 2.1ng/ml and his prostate feels smoothly enlarged.

64) An 84-year-old male is found to have adenocarcinoma of the prostate with metastases in the pelvis and spine. He has a history of ischaemic heart disease with cardiac stents *in situ*. He lives alone at home and carries out all his daily self-care independently but is unable to walk up a flight of stairs without taking a GTN spray.

65) A 68-year-old male is under investigation for suspected prostate cancer. His PSA is 7.0ng/ml and imaging is suggestive of a tumour in the anterior prostate.

Glasgow Coma Scale

a.	1.	e.	12.
b.	5.	f.	9.
c.	8.	g.	3.
d.	15.	h.	10.

Match the description of the patient with the correct GCS score.

66) A young male found to have an extradural haematoma on a CT scan is opening his eyes when you say hello. He is slurring his speech and you are unable to make out any clear words. He responds to pain by pulling away the part of his body affected.

67) A female patient presents with a sudden onset occipital headache. This is the worst headache she has ever had and her neck is extremely stiff also. She has vomited several times. She opens her eyes as normal and is able to tell you what has happened to her and where she is now. She is able to stand and walk in a straight line when you ask her to.

68) A male is brought into the emergency department resus following a major RTC. He was riding a motorbike at the time. On arrival his eyes are closed and do not open despite the best efforts of the medical team. He makes no sounds and makes no motor effort when prompted, nor when painful stimuli are applied. His vital signs, however, remain within normal limits.

69) An elderly male presents to the emergency department following a fall and head injury. He has a large laceration over his forehead and a CT scan shows a large subdural haematoma. He opens his eyes in response to pain, he is talking to you but sounds confused and he pulls his arm away when painful stimulus is applied to it.

70) A female is found collapsed at the bus station. She is known to the alcohol misuse clinic and there is concern that she frequently falls and injures herself. She appears to have hit her head. She is responding to voice by opening her eyes and following commands. She is talking but is swearing profusely at staff and is unable to correctly identify objects with the appropriate words.

Treatment of vascular disease

a.	Medical management.	e.	Embolectomy.
b.	Graduated compression stockings.	f.	Urgent open repair.
c.	Sclerotherapy.	g.	No treatment required.
d.	Endovascular aneurysm repair.	h.	Carotid endarterectomy.

Match the description with the most appropriate treatment option.

71) A 66-year-old male presents to the emergency department with retrosternal chest pain which is sudden onset and tearing in nature. The pain radiates to his arms. A CT of the chest shows the presence of an aortic dissection involving the descending aorta distal to the left subclavian artery.

72) A 60-year-old female with atrial fibrillation presents to the emergency department with pain, pallor and absent pulses in her left leg. The consultant suspects she has acute limb ischaemia secondary to atrial fibrillation.

73) A 34-year-old female asks her primary care doctor to review several prominent veins on her left calf. On examination, she has multiple varicosities and a positive tourniquet test. The patient would like to opt for medical management rather than surgery.

74) A 72-year-old female presents with a 3-month history of cramping pain on walking short distances. She could walk 800 metres 12 months ago but now can only walk 400 metres before she gets pain. On examination, peripheral pulses are reduced on the left and the limb is cooler compared with the right. There is no sign of gangrene, necrosis or ulceration.

75) A 45-year-old female attends the vascular clinic following a referral from her primary care doctor. She has numerous varicose veins on her right leg and the patient would like to be evaluated for surgery rather than further medical treatment.

Upper limb X-ray findings

a.	Colles' fracture.	e.	Galeazzi fracture.
b.	Smith's fracture.	f.	Monteggia fracture.
c.	Bennett's fracture.	g.	Radial head fracture.
d.	Volar Barton's fracture.	h.	Boxer's fracture.

Match the description of the X-ray with the most likely diagnosis.

76) A proximal ulna fracture with disruption of the proximal radioulnar joint.

77) A distal radius fracture with dorsal angulation.

78) A distal third radial fracture with disruption of the distal radio-ulna joint.

79) An intra-articular base of thumb fracture.

80) A fracture of the head of the fifth metacarpal with volar angulation.

ABG normal values

a.	11-13.	e.	7.35-7.45.
b.	15-18.	f.	-2 to +2.
c.	22-28.	g.	7.39-7.49.
d.	17-25.	h.	12-16.

Match the ABG result with the most likely diagnosis.

81) What is a normal pH?

82) What is the normal PaO_2 in kPa?

83) What is the normal bicarbonate in mmol/L?

84) What is the normal base excess in mmol/L?

85) What is a normal anion gap in mmol/L?

Facial pain

a.	Acute sinusitis.	e.	Parotid tumour.
b.	Chronic sinusitis.	f.	Sinusitis.
c.	Mumps.	g.	Trauma.
d.	Nasopharyngeal tumour.	h.	Trigeminal neuralgia.

Match the description of the patient with the most likely diagnosis.

86) A 9-year-old boy is sent to see the school nurse because he has painful swelling next to his ear and feels unwell.

87) A 48-year-old female is taking carbamazepine to treat pain in her face.

88) A 67-year-old retired carpenter sees the primary care doctor with pain in the middle of his face and a blocked nose, which he has had for 3 weeks. He says only the left nostril is blocked.

89) A 67-year-old retired teacher sees the primary care doctor with pain in the middle of his face and a blocked nose, which he has had for 3 days. Both nostrils are blocked.

90) A 31-year-old female has pain in her forehead and a cough. She feels unwell and her temperature is 37.9°C.

Management of cancer

a. Combined chemotherapy/ radiotherapy.

b. Chemotherapy only.

c. Radiotherapy only.

d. Brachytherapy only.

e. Bowel resection.

f. Lung resection.

g. Whipple's procedure.

h. No action needed.

Choose the next step of the management plan from the above list.

91) A 65-year-old male has a colonoscopy as a result of a positive faecal occult blood test. He is found to have localised colorectal cancer in the descending colon. He has a performance status of 0.

92) A 67-year-old male presents with a lump in his neck. Biopsy notes a squamous cell carcinoma of the tonsil. He undergoes an operation and is suitable for radical therapy.

93) A 78-year-old smoker presents with haemoptysis. She is found on biopsy to have a small cell lung cancer anatomically close to the mediastinum.

94) A 57-year-old male is found to have pancreatic cancer. What is the only curative management that could be offered to this patient who is fit and well otherwise?

95) A 45-year-old male finds a unilateral testicular lump. After investigation he is shown to have a metastatic non-seminomatous germ cell tumour which has metastasised to his lung. He is planned for an orchidectomy. What curative treatment should be offered next?

Ocular pathology and disease

a.	Central retinal artery occlusion.	e.	ARMD — wet.
b.	Central retinal vein occlusion.	f.	Diabetic maculopathy.
c.	Retinopathy of prematurity.	g.	ARMD — dry.
d.	Proliferative diabetic retinopathy.	h.	Hypertensive retinopathy.

Match the description of the patient with the most likely diagnosis.

96) A 20-year-old Type 1 diabetic is pregnant with her second child. She has noticed increasing visual loss. Fundoscopy reveals cotton wool spots, exudate and new retinal vessel formation.

97) A 52-year-old male smoker presents to his primary care doctor with gradual changes in his vision. On examination, he has a generalised arteriole narrowing with irregular points of focal constriction.

98) An 82-year-old female presents to her primary care doctor with a progressive loss of central vision which has made reading difficult. She denies any pain or trauma. On examination, she has a central scotoma and visual distortion; peripheral vision is intact. Pupillary examination is normal. Fundoscopy shows retinal thickening with new vessels at this site and evidence of haemorrhage.

99) A 45-year-old male with known hypertension attends with sudden painless loss of vision in his right eye. On examination, he has a reduced visual acuity on the right and fundoscopy shows flame haemorrhages, venous dilatation, a swollen optic disc and macular oedema.

100) A 2-week-old neonate is seen for regular eye screening as he was delivered at 30 weeks. Following delivery, he required prolonged supplementary oxygenation. Fundoscopy notes a retinal ridge with blood vessels growing up to this point.

Drug overdose

a.	Tricyclic antidepressant.	e.	Paracetamol.
b.	Aspirin.	f.	Benzodiazepine.
c.	Lithium.	g.	Opiates.
d.	Beta blockers.	h.	Antifreeze.

Match the description below with the most likely causative substance.

101) Ataxia, coarse tremor and dysarthria.

102) Abdominal pain and ringing in the ears. A venous blood gas shows a respiratory alkalosis.

103) This substance can be reversed using flumazenil.

104) Reduced GCS, respiratory rate of 4 breaths per minute and pinpoint pupils.

105) Overdose of this substance is the most common cause of acute liver failure in the United Kingdom.

Immunisation schedule

a. DTaP/IPV/Hib/HepB.   e. HPV.
b. MenB.   f. MenACWY.
c. PCV.   g. MMR.
d. Rotavirus.   h. Td/IPV.

Match the appropriate vaccination with each age below.

106) 8 weeks, 12 weeks, and 16 weeks.

107) 1 year, and 3 years 4 months.

108) 14 years.

109) 8 and 12 weeks.

110) 12-13 years.

Vaginal infections

a.   *Candida albicans.*
b.   *Chlamydia trachomatis.*
c.   *Trichomonas vaginalis.*
d.   Herpes simplex virus.

e.   Human papilloma virus.
f.   *Neisseria gonorrhoeae.*
g.   *Gardnerella spp.*
h.   *Treponema pallidum.*

Match the patient with the most likely causative organism.

111) A 50-year-old female presents with a painless lesion of the vulva which has a small ulcer forming at the centre.

112) A 19-year-old female presents with a history of unprotected sex 2 weeks previously and on swabs a Gram-negative diplococcus is cultured.

113) A 24-year-old female presents with increased vaginal discharge and clue cells are seen on microscopy.

114) A 32-year-old female presents with several painful ulcers on the vulva.

115) An 18-year-old female presents to a genito-urinary medicine clinic following a trip to Magaluf for routine STI screening. Swabs show a flagellated protozoa.

Changes in pigmentation

a. Neurofibromatosis.
b. Pityriasis versicolor.
c. Vitiligo.
d. Albinism.

e. Amiodarone.
f. Addison's disease.
g. Haemochromatosis.
h. Tuberous sclerosis.

Match the description to the most likely cause of symptoms.

116) A 6-year-old male is seen by a geneticist. He has a genetic disorder which has manifested with mild learning difficulties and multiple light-brown flat macules.

117) Blue-grey discolouration associated with thyroid abnormalities.

118) A 23-year-old female with a background of Type 1 diabetes attends her primary care doctor with a history of nausea, loss of appetite and abdominal pain. On examination, there is hyperpigmentation of her buccal mucosa and she has a postural drop in her blood pressure.

119) May present in childhood with seizures. Ash leaf macules are often found on dermatological examination.

120) A 28-year-old female with hypothyroidism presents with bilateral symmetrical hypopigmented patches.

Pharmacological mechanisms of action

a. Vitamin K antagonist.
b. COX-1 inhibitor.
c. Non-selective COX inhibitor.
d. $P2Y_{12}$ ADP inhibitor.

e. Beta-2 antagonist.
f. Beta-2 agonist.
g. H_2 antagonist.
h. H^+/K^+ ATPase inhibitor.

Match the appropriate drug with the correct mechanism of action.

121) Proton pump inhibitors such as lansoprazole or omeprazole.

122) Salbutamol.

123) Clopidogrel.

124) Aspirin.

125) Warfarin.

Antibiotic mechanisms of action

a. Co-amoxiclav.
b. Daptomycin.
c. Polymyxins.
d. Rifampicin.

e. Vancomycin.
f. Gentamicin.
g. Trimethoprim.
h. Erythromycin.

Match the appropriate drug with the correct mechanism of action.

126) A beta-lactam antibiotic with potassium clavulanate which inhibits cell wall synthesis.

127) Inhibits protein synthesis by binding to the 50S subunit.

128) Inhibits protein synthesis by binding to the 30S subunit.

129) Inhibits folate synthesis.

130) Inhibits cell wall synthesis and is used in the oral form in the treatment of *Clostridium difficile* infection.

Statistical definitions

a.   Sensitivity.
b.   Specificity.
c.   Number needed to treat.
d.   Positive predicted value.

e.   Negative predicted value.
f.   Null hypothesis.
g.   Odds ratio.
h.   Prevalence.

Match the appropriate definition with the correct phrase.

131) The percentage of people with the disease that will have a positive test result.

132) The percentage of people without the disease that will have a negative test result.

133) The chance that a patient receiving a positive result will actually have the disease.

134) The chance that a patient receiving a negative result will not actually have the disease.

135) The proportion of a population with a disease at a specific point in time.

Ethical principles

a.   Autonomy.   e.   Deontology.

b.   Beneficence.   f.   Virtue.

c.   Justice.   g.   Consequentialism.

d.   Non-maleficence.   h.   Paternalism.

Match the appropriate drug with the correct mechanism of action.

136) The main concern is to respect rights and duties rather than the consequences of an action.

137) This is concerned with the consequences of a particular behaviour. Utilitarianism is the most common form of this theory.

138) This de-emphasises rules and consequences of a particular act and focuses on the character of the person performing the act. It can be culturally specific and ignores community and social dimensions.

139) This is the obligation to avoid causing harm to another person.

140) This is the idea of ensuring decisions are made by the individual and are not decided on the patient's behalf by another person.

Chapter 3

Practice paper 3
QUESTIONS

Short answer questions

1) A 65-year-old male presents to the emergency department with recurrent severe episodes of cardiac chest pain. These initially only occurred on exertion, but now occur at rest. There are no acute ECG changes and no troponin rise. The admitting team suspects unstable angina.

a. Name two mechanisms of action of angina medication used for symptom relief. 2 marks

b. Specify the gold standard test for investigating coronary artery disease. 1 mark

c. Name four medication classes used in secondary prevention. 4 marks

d. Name the surgical intervention used in patients that are unsuitable for primary percutaneous coronary intervention. 1 mark

e. Name two complications of this surgical intervention. 2 marks

2) A 53-year-old male presents with pleuritic chest pain and shortness of breath. The pain was sudden and there is no history of trauma. He is very tall with an arm span greater than height. He has a past medical history of lens dislocation. A chest X-ray confirms a 5cm pneumothorax.

a. What is the most appropriate treatment in this patient?   1 mark
b. Name three underlying lung diseases that can predispose to a   3 marks
    spontaneous pneumothorax.
c. State three signs that suggest a tension pneumothorax.   3 marks
d. From where is the size of a pneumothorax measured?   1 mark
e. Name two surgical interventions that could be considered should   2 marks
    there be reoccurrence of the pneumothorax.

3) A 65-year-old male presents with a 3-month history of dysphagia to solids and liquids. He is a current smoker. He has noticed a 2-stone unintentional weight loss over the past 3 months.

a. What is the underlying diagnosis?   1 mark
b. State four risk factors for this condition.   2 marks
c. Define three other causes of dysphagia.   3 marks
d. Give two investigations that should be considered.   2 marks
e. State two management options for this patient.   2 marks

4) You are the doctor on-call and are clerking a referral from a local primary care doctor, who refers a patient with cerebral palsy and a long-term catheter with abnormal blood test results and reduced urine output. Whilst he has some communication and learning difficulties, he expresses pain when palpated in the suprapubic region. You suspect a post-renal cause for the blood test results.

a. State how post-renal AKI occurs and provide one example.   2 marks

b. Give two simple bedside interventions you could perform to   2 marks
    investigate or treat the cause of reduced urine output.

c. Give three biochemical markers raised in acute infection.   3 marks

d. Give two contraindications to suprapubic catheterisation.   2 marks

e. Name one analgesic which is inappropriate for use in AKI.   1 mark

5) A 22-year-old female presents to her primary care doctor
    feeling lethargic and mentioning a 3-week history of
    excessive thirst and frequent urination. The primary care
    doctor is concerned about Type 1 diabetes.

a. Which cells in the pancreas are affected in diabetes?   2 marks

b. Name one gene commonly mutated in Type 1 diabetes.   2 marks

c. Name one antibody to differentiate Type 1 and Type 2 diabetes.   1 mark

d. State the value for diabetes diagnosis on a glucose tolerance test.   2 marks

e. Name three potential complications of Type 1 diabetes.   3 marks

6) A 49-year-old woman is admitted with loss of sensation
    and weakness in her left leg. She has no past medical
    history aside from an episode of optic neuritis 2 years ago.
    On examination, she has increased tone and brisk reflexes
    in her left leg. Power is 0/5 and light touch sensation is
    absent. You suspect she may have multiple sclerosis.

a. Describe the pathophysiological process responsible.   2 marks

b. She notices that her symptoms are worse when she gets out of a hot   1 mark
    bath. What is the name used to describe this?

c. Name two investigations that could be performed and the findings   4 marks
    you would expect.

d. What class of drug can be given for the acute attack?   1 mark

e. Name two drugs which may affect disease progression in relapsing   2 marks
    remitting multiple sclerosis.

7) The phrase microangiopathic haemolytic anaemia (MAHA) encompass several different disease processes including haemolytic uraemic syndrome (HUS) and thrombotic thrombocytopenic purpura (TTP)

a. Describe the process which results in haemolysis. 1 mark
b. What three characteristic symptoms are seen in HUS? 3 marks
c. What system is typically affected in individuals with TTP? 2 marks
d. What can be seen on the blood film of people with MAHA? 2 marks
e. What is the antibody associated with TTP targeted against? 2 marks

8) A 36-year-old female visits her primary care doctor feeling feverish with chills, myalgia, a headache and cough for the last couple of days. She has been unable to go to work and has done nothing other than lie in bed since becoming unwell. On examination, she is pyrexial at 38.9°C, BP 125/90mmHg, HR 88 bpm, RR 18 breaths per minute, saturations 98% on air; auscultation of the chest is unremarkable. You suspect she has influenza.

a. Give three other common viral causes of coryzal symptoms. 3 marks
b. Name two surface antigens present on the influenza A virus. 2 marks
c. The primary care doctor is concerned about a major and sudden change in the surface antigens in the virus. What is this phenomenon? 1 mark
d. Specify six vaccine preventable diseases other than influenza. 3 marks
e. State one antiviral drug that can reduce the duration of symptoms in influenza. 1 mark

9) A 50-year-old female is referred to the rheumatology clinic with acid reflux and problems swallowing food. These symptoms have been present for the past month and are getting worse. She has also been experiencing painful fingers on exposure to the cold. Her fingers turn white and are acutely painful; this resolves on warming and her fingers go transiently red before settling to normal. She has a history of hypertension and hypothyroidism and does not smoke or drink alcohol. After further history and investigation, the rheumatologist diagnoses limited scleroderma with systemic involvement (CREST syndrome).

a. Specify two autoantibodies associated with this condition. 2 marks
b. State three skin changes you may find on examination. 3 marks
c. Name two pulmonary complications from this disease. 2 marks
d. Identify one drug class and example that is used to treat Raynaud's disease. 2 marks
e. What treatment could you offer for her reflux symptoms? 1 mark

10) A 54-year-old female presents to the emergency department with a 12-hour history of right upper quadrant pain. It started following eating her breakfast and has continued throughout the day. She describes the pain as colicky in nature. Blood results show a raised white cell count and raised CRP.

a. Name four differentials for the above patient. 2 marks
b. State four initial investigations that would be useful. 2 marks
c. What is the underlying diagnosis? 1 mark
d. Give two initial management options for this patient. 2 marks
e. Name three complications of this patient's condition. 3 marks

11) A 67-year-old male has had a reversal of a Hartmann's procedure 7 days ago. The Hartmann's was initially done for severe diverticulitis. The surgical registrar is concerned there may be an anastomotic leak because the patient has developed fever and abdominal pain.

a.	Suggest two features that may be found on examination.	2 marks
b.	What investigation would be used to confirm the diagnosis?	1 mark
c.	Give two risk factors for an anastomotic leak.	2 marks
d.	Give three other possible complications of stoma reversal.	3 marks
e.	State two management strategies for this patient.	2 marks

12) A 60-year-old female presents to her primary care doctor with a breast lump. She last had screening 2 years ago, which was normal. You take a history and inform her that you will need to examine her. She consents to this.

a.	Name the four stages of assessing capacity to consent.	2 marks
b.	What must you ask her before the examination begins?	1 mark
c.	Describe in four stages how you carry out a breast examination.	4 marks
d.	State two other areas that you must examine.	2 marks
e.	The examination is normal; what would you do now?	1 mark

13) A 31-year-old male has tightness of the foreskin that causes pain when he has an erection. He reports that his foreskin has always been tight but over the last few years he has been unable to retract it.

a.	State the difference between phimosis and paraphimosis.	2 marks
b.	Is phimosis always pathological?	1 mark
c.	How should paraphimosis be managed?	3 marks
d.	What is priapism?	1 mark
e.	What causes priapism?	3 marks

14) A 56-year-old female presents to the emergency department following a seizure. The seizure was a generalised tonic clonic seizure which self-resolved after around 3 minutes. The family states they have been encouraging her to visit the doctor for some time as she has had progressive weakness of one arm for several months and been complaining of headaches. They also state her personality has changed steadily over recent months. You suspect a primary brain tumour.

a.   What is the most common CNS tumour?   1 mark
b.   Name two other type of CNS tumours.   2 marks
c.   In which lobe is this tumour most likely located?   1 mark
d.   Specify three treatments that may be used for CNS tumours.   3 marks
e.   What is meant by a high-grade tumour?   3 marks

15) An 80-year-old male visits his primary care doctor with a pain in his right leg after walking that feels crampy in nature; the pain starts after walking approximately 600 metres. He could walk 900 metres 12 months ago before he felt this pain. The pain resolves at rest and with simple analgesia. He is concerned regarding his decrease in exercise tolerance.

a.   What is the underlying diagnosis?   1 mark
b.   Specify three risk factors for this condition.   3 marks
c.   Name two possible treatment options for this patient.   2 marks
d.   The patient returns to clinic after 12 months with a reduced walking   2 marks
     distance of 50 yards, pain at rest and at night. State two investigations
     that should be arranged.
e.   Name two treatment options for these new symptoms.   2 marks

16) A 56-year-old female attends the emergency department with a 2-day history of back pain which is shooting down her leg. She saw her primary care doctor this morning and he was concerned that she hasn't passed urine all day because she had not felt the need. On examination, the power in her lower limbs is normal but she has some reduced sensation in the L5 distribution on the right.

a.	Define sciatica and give two potential causes.	3 marks
b.	List four red flags for back pain.	2 marks
c.	Define cauda equina syndrome and the potential sequalae.	2 marks
d.	State two features of the history or examination that lead you to suspect cauda equina syndrome.	2 marks
e.	How will you further investigate this pain?	1 mark

17) You are called by the nursing staff as the laboratory has phoned through a patient's haemoglobin level; it is currently 64g/L and the patient has noted some shortness of breath and fatigue. A 2-unit blood transfusion is given and the haemoglobin the following day has risen to 84g/L.

a.	What type of fluid is blood?	1 mark
b.	Explain the term permissive hypotension.	2 marks
c.	Name four types of transfusion reaction.	4 marks
d.	What two electrolyte abnormalities may occur from a large-volume blood transfusion?	1 mark
e.	If the patient was a Jehovah's Witness, name two treatments which would be acceptable to the patient.	2 marks

18) A 67-year-old retired bus driver is referred to ENT with hearing loss and pain in his right ear. On examination, he has a vesicular rash on the pinna. He also has a right-sided facial weakness which includes the forehead. The ENT registrar suspects Ramsay Hunt syndrome.

a.	Describe the pathology of Ramsay Hunt syndrome.	2 marks
b.	Name two more possible features of the syndrome.	2 marks
c.	Name two medical treatments that can be given.	2 marks
d.	Name two treatments that may help with symptoms.	2 marks
e.	What is the prognosis?	2 marks

19) A 67-year-old male presents to his primary care doctor with weight loss and dysphagia. The primary care doctor is concerned regarding malignancy and refers him for an urgent oesophageal gastroduodenoscopy (OGD).

a.	List two other red flag symptoms for oesophageal cancer.	2 marks
b.	What anaemia are you likely to see in malignancy?	1 mark
c.	What condition is pre-cancerous when it occurs in the oesophagus? Describe the pathology seen and the underlying cause.	3 marks
d.	He has significant odynophagia and is malnourished. What procedure may be offered to him and what may he be at risk of if he begins feeding after a prolonged period of starvation?	2 marks
e.	The patient returns to clinic 2 months later with a hoarse voice. State the likely cause.	2 marks

20) A 7-year-old female attends her primary care doctor with bilaterally red itchy eyes which started 3 days ago; it initially started in her left eye but now both eyes are affected. Her father says he noticed her eyes were sticky and she complained of a gritty sensation. On examination, you note bilateral mild chemosis, a purulent discharge and mild preauricular lymphadenopathy.

a. What is the diagnosis?   1 mark
b. Specify four other common causes of a red eye.   2 marks
c. Name three extraocular barriers to infection.   3 marks
d. Name the most common viral and two common bacterial causes of   3 marks
   this condition.
e. State one difference between bacterial and viral forms of this   1 mark
   condition.

21) A 76-year-old male is admitted to hospital with increasing confusion and visual hallucinations. Clinical examination reveals parkinsonism and a delirium screen is negative. A collateral history is obtained from the family who report fluctuating confusion for 1 year and believe he has been responding to visual hallucinations for several months. The medical team suspect this is dementia with Lewy bodies.

a. State two other features of dementia with Lewy bodies.   2 marks
b. What triad of symptoms is present in motor parkinsonism?   3 marks
c. Give three other causes of dementia.   3 marks
d. State one medication that should be offered first-line in mild to   1 mark
   moderate dementia with Lewy bodies.
e. What neurological disorder is described: features are progressive   1 mark
   dementia, parkinsonism, postural instability, dysphagia and difficulty
   with eye movements particularly in vertical gaze?

22) A 3-year-old child has presented with recurrent productive coughs and has required multiple courses of antibiotics. As a newborn, she was tested for cystic fibrosis and was found to be positive.

a. Why has she developed recurrent respiratory infections?   1 mark

b. What is the most common gene mutation that causes this condition, and what protein does this gene code for?   2 marks

c. Name three organs significantly affected in this condition.   3 marks

d. What test is frequently used to diagnose this condition?   1 mark

e. Give three management options used in this condition.   3 marks

23) A woman presents to her primary care doctor at 8 weeks postpartum complaining of low mood and being more tearful since the birth of her daughter.

a. What is the incidence of postnatal depression?   1 mark

b. Name five risk factors for developing postnatal depression.   5 marks

c. State two antidepressant classes used in breastfeeding.   2 marks

d. Which other mental health condition occurs postpartum?   1 mark

e. Which pre-existing mental disorder causes the highest proportion of postnatal depression amongst its sufferers?   1 mark

24) A 28-year-old female presents to her primary care doctor complaining of weight loss and diarrhoea. On examination, her pulse is regular at 102 bpm; she has a fine tremor and appears anxious, and there is a palpable small, firm diffuse goitre. She is normally fit and well, and she takes the combined oral contraceptive pill only. You clinically suspect that she may have thyroid disease.

a. State three dermatological findings in hyperthyroidism.   3 marks
b. Give three dermatological findings in hypothyroidism.   3 marks
c. The following results are received; what is the diagnosis?   2 marks

TSH: <0.02mIU/L (0.27-4.2mIU/L)
Free T4: 28.0pmol/L (12.0-22.0pmol/L)
TPO antibodies: positive
Thyroglobulin antibodies: positive

d. Name one medication that you would commence.   1 mark
e. She later presents to the emergency department with a temperature 1 mark
    of 38.5°C, an irregular heart rate of 138 bpm, confusion and diarrhoea
    and vomiting. On examination, you find no evidence of an acute
    infection. What is the most likely diagnosis?

25) 800 patients take part in a study to assess the accuracy of
    a new screening test for diabetes mellitus. 400 patients
    were known to have diabetes and 400 patients enrolled
    did not have diabetes. 340 of the known diabetic patients
    had a positive result using the new test and 100 of the
    patients without diabetes tested positive for diabetes
    using the new test.

a. Calculate the sensitivity for the above test.   2 marks
b. Calculate the specificity for the above test.   2 marks
c. Calculate the positive predicted value for the above test.   2 marks
d. Calculate the negative predicted value for the above test.   2 marks
e. Calculate the prevalence of the condition for the above test.   2 marks

26) A 32-year-old female presents to the emergency department with a 3-hour history of a severe unilateral headache. The patient describes the pain as severe and burning. The pain is localised around the eye and temple. On examination, you note a red and watery eye with ptosis and drooping of the left eyelid. She is also sweating profusely and feels as if her sinuses are blocked.

a. What is the underlying diagnosis? 1 mark

b. Name four red flag features in a headache history that would necessitate urgent investigation. 4 marks

c. List two first-line treatments for this patient. 2 marks

d. State one prophylactic treatment that can be used in this patient. 1 mark

e. Give two possible triggers for a cluster headache. 2 marks

27) A 70-year-old male presents with loss of vision in his left eye for more than 30 minutes. He is seen in the emergency department 60 minutes after symptom presentation. On examination, you note cortical blindness and a contralateral homonymous hemianopia. He does not have any weakness or gait disturbance.

a. What is the most likely diagnosis? 1 mark

b. Which vessel is most likely to be affected? 1 mark

c. Name three relative contraindications to thrombolysis. 3 marks

d. Name three absolute contraindications to thrombolysis. 3 marks

e. Name two classes of drugs used in the secondary prevention of stroke. 2 marks

28) A 30-year-old female presents to her primary care doctor with a 5-day history of jaundice following a respiratory tract infection. She has had similar symptoms following periods of illness previously. Liver function tests show a raised unconjugated bilirubin. The primary care doctor arranges for several tests to be carried out; however, 2 days following the consultation the patient contacts her doctor to inform her the jaundice has resolved.

a.   What is the underlying diagnosis?   1 mark
b.   How is jaundice classified and provide two examples for each?   3 marks
c.   Describe urine and stool findings that would be seen in this patient.   2 marks
d.   Which enzyme is likely to be reduced or deficient in this patient? 1 mark
e.   Name three complications of jaundice.   3 marks

29) A 62-year-old male is reviewed in the cardiology clinic for extertional dyspnoea. On examination, you note a murmur best heard at the left sternal edge and a collapsing pulse. You suspect a diagnosis of aortic regurgitation.

a.   State three other symptoms that the patient may experience.   3 marks
b.   What type of murmur would be heard on auscultation?   2 marks
c.   List two associated findings that may be seen in this patient.   2 marks
d.   State one investigation that can be requested to further assess this   1 mark
     patient.
e.   Name two conditions that predisposes patients to the above   2 marks
     diagnosis.

30) A 58-year-old female presents to the neurology clinic with a stooping gait. She is a typist and has found that her dexterity is reduced. On examination, you note a resting tremor in her right hand, reduced arm swing, difficultly in performing rapid fine movements, increased tone and cogwheel rigidity on the right.

a. What is the most likely diagnosis in this patient?   1 mark
b. Give three further signs or symptoms that may be present.   3 marks
c. State the neurotransmitter and location which is deficient in this condition.   2 marks
d. Name two classes of drugs that can be used to treat this condition.   2 marks
e. List two complications associated with long-term treatment of dopamine replacement therapy.   2 marks

31) A 62-year-old male presents with central crushing chest pain radiating to his arm. An ECG is performed which shows ST segment elevation in leads II, III and aVF with reciprocal ST depression in aVL

a. What is the underlying diagnosis?   1 mark
b. Which coronary artery is most likely to be occluded?   1 mark
c. State three immediate management options for this patient.   3 marks
d. Give one definitive management for this patient.   1 mark
e. Name four complications of a myocardial infarction.   4 marks

32) An 18-year-old female presents to her primary care doctor with increasing shortness of breath and chest tightness. She finds that her breathlessness is worst in the morning. On examination, you note a mild expiratory wheeze and normal oxygen saturations.

a. What is the underlying diagnosis?   1 mark
b. State three common triggers for this condition.   3 marks
c. What type of pattern would be seen on spirometry assessment?   1 mark
d. State the first-line management for this patient.   1 mark
e. Describe the stepwise approach that can be used if the patient is not   4 marks
   well controlled using first-line management.

33) A 43-year-old male presents to his primary care doctor with a change in bowel habit. He is referred for a colonoscopy which shows a large mass projecting into the lumen of the colon. His father was diagnosed with colorectal cancer at the age of 45 years.

a. What is the underlying diagnosis?   1 mark
b. Name four factors that must be fulfilled in the Amsterdam II Criteria   4 marks
   for this diagnosis to be accepted.
c. Name two other genetic syndromes associated with the development   2 marks
   of bowel cancer.
d. What genetic abnormality may be present in this patient?   1 mark
e. Name two other tumours that are associated with the patient's   2 marks
   diagnosis.

34) A 21-year-old male presents to his primary care doctor with a painless lump in his neck, that has been present for over 4 weeks. The doctor is concerned that the patient may have lymphoma.

a. List the three B-symptoms associated with lymphoma. 3 marks
b. State two signs of examination that may be present. 2 marks
c. How could the diagnosis of lymphoma be confirmed? 1 mark
d. List three staging investigations for this patient. 3 marks
e. What is the name of the staging system used in Hodgkin's lymphoma? 1 mark

35) An 18-year-old male presents to his primary care doctor with a 4-day history of haematuria. The doctor undertakes several investigations which note haematuria, proteinuria, hypertension and uraemia.

a. What is the underlying diagnosis? 1 mark
b. State five causes of this condition. 5 marks
c. Name two investigations to help provide a definitive diagnosis. 2 marks
d. List one indication for dialysis in this patient. 1 mark
e. If auto-antibodies to type IV collagen were found, what would be the underlying diagnosis? 1 mark

36) A 54-year-old male presents to the emergency room with a 48-hour history of severe epigastric pain radiating to the back. He has a past medical history of heavy alcohol use. On examination, he is tender in the epigastrium.

a. What is the most likely underlying cause? 1 mark
b. List four other causes of pancreatitis. 4 marks
c. Name one blood test that would confirm the diagnosis of pancreatitis. 1 mark
d. State two early complications of this condition. 2 marks
e. State two late complications of this condition. 2 marks

37) A 50-year-old male presents to his primary care doctor as his wife has noticed that a mole on his arm has changed in appearance over the past 6 weeks. On examination, you note an asymmetrical pigmented lesion with a rough appearance and irregular border. The patient is seen by a dermatologist who diagnoses a stage 2A malignant melanoma.

a. You discuss with the medical student about the 'ABCDE' approach; describe how the factors are used to examine a changing pigmented lesion.   5 marks

b. List two risk factors for this condition.   2 marks

c. Name one subtype for the above diagnosis.   1 mark

d. State the most common genetic mutation associated with this condition.   1 mark

e. Name one treatment option for this patient.   1 mark

38) A 28-year-old female attends for a regular cervical screening. She receives the result 4 weeks later which reveals cervical intra-epithelial neoplasia 2.

a. Name three risk factors for cervical cancer.   3 marks

b. What is the most common organism associated with cervical cancer?   1 mark

c. Name two high-risk subtypes of this organism associated with cervical cancer.   2 marks

d. List three pieces of advice you would give to minimise the risk of cervical cancer.   3 marks

e. State which treatment option is most appropriate for this patient.   1 mark

39) A 3-year-old child presents to the emergency room with a prolonged fever and multiple systemic symptoms. The admitting doctor is concerned that the child has Kawasaki's disease.

a.	List the five diagnostic criteria for this disease.	5 marks
b.	State one investigation for this patient.	1 mark
c.	State one differential diagnosis.	1 mark
d.	Name two treatment options for this disease.	2 marks
e.	Name one complication of this disease.	1 mark

40) A 24-year-old male presents to the emergency room with a 2-day history of headache, fever and vomiting. On examination, he has a non-blanching rash, neck stiffness, fever and photophobia.

a.	What is the underlying diagnosis?	2 marks
b.	What is the most likely causative organism?	1 mark
c.	State three findings on the lumbar puncture.	3 marks
d.	Name two findings in the lumbar puncture if a fungal organism was responsible for the patient's symptoms.	2 marks
e.	Name two findings in the lumbar puncture if there was a viral cause for the patient's symptoms.	2 marks

Chapter 4

Abdominal X-ray
QUESTIONS

Interpretation questions

Please interpret the following abdominal X-rays shown overleaf:

Abdominal X-ray 1
Abdominal X-ray 2
Abdominal X-ray 3
Abdominal X-ray 4
Abdominal X-ray 5

Abdominal X-ray question 1:

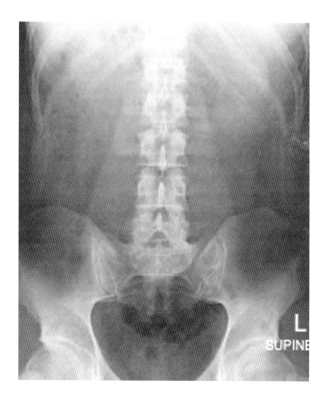

Image quality: _____

Air: _____

Bowels: _____

Calcifications: _____

Densities: _____

Everything else: _____

Diagnosis: _____

Abdominal X-ray question 2:

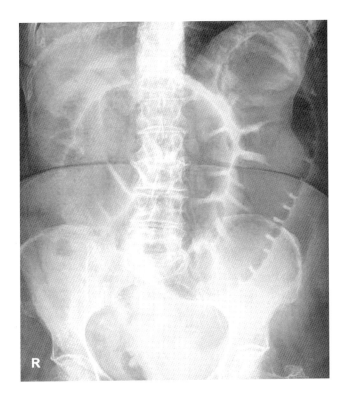

Image quality: _____

Air: _____

Bowels: _____

Calcifications: _____

Densities: _____

Everything else: _____

Diagnosis: _____

Abdominal X-ray question 3:

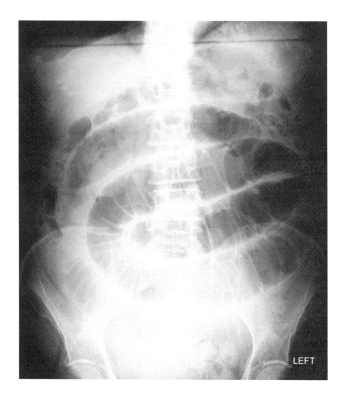

Image quality: _____

Air: _____

Bowels: _____

Calcifications: _____

Densities: _____

Everything else: _____

Diagnosis: _____

Abdominal X-ray question 4:

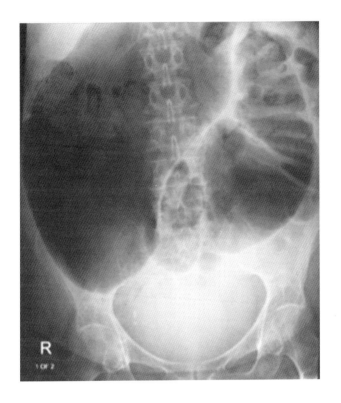

Image quality: _____

Air: _____

Bowels: _____

Calcifications: _____

Densities: _____

Everything else: _____

Diagnosis: _____

Abdominal X-ray question 5:

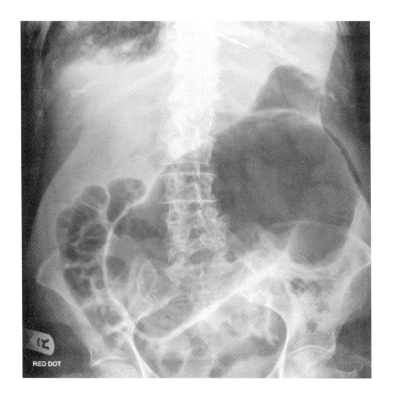

Image quality: _____

Air: _____

Bowels: _____

Calcifications: _____

Densities: _____

Everything else: _____

Diagnosis: _____

Chapter 5

Chest X-ray
QUESTIONS

Interpretation questions

Please interpret the following chest X-rays shown overleaf:

Chest X-ray 1
Chest X-ray 2
Chest X-ray 3
Chest X-ray 4
Chest X-ray 5
Chest X-ray 6
Chest X-ray 7

Chest X-ray question 1:

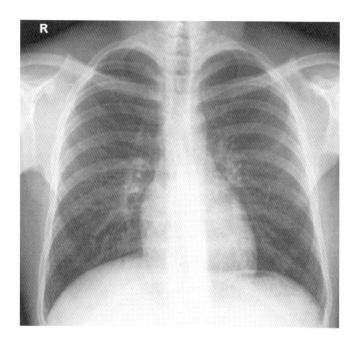

Image quality: _____

Airway: _____

Breathing: _____

Circulation: _____

Diaphragm: _____

Everything else: _____

Diagnosis: _____

Chest X-ray question 2:

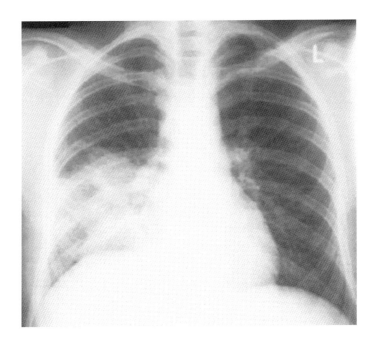

Image quality: _____

Airway: _____

Breathing: _____

Circulation: _____

Diaphragm: _____

Everything else: _____

Diagnosis: _____

Chest X-ray question 3:

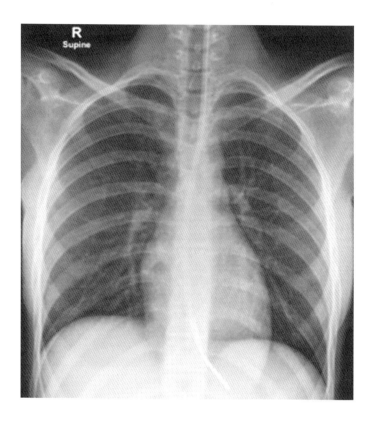

Image quality: _____

Airway: _____

Breathing: _____

Circulation: _____

Diaphragm: _____

Everything else: _____

Diagnosis: _____

Chest X-ray question 4:

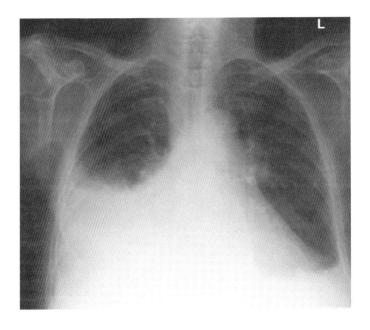

Image quality: _____

Airway: _____

Breathing: _____

Circulation: _____

Diaphragm: _____

Everything else: _____

Diagnosis: _____

Chest X-ray question 5:

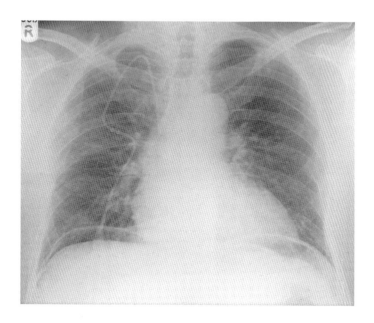

Image quality: _____

Airway: _____

Breathing: _____

Circulation: _____

Diaphragm: _____

Everything else: _____

Diagnosis: _____

Chest X-ray question 6:

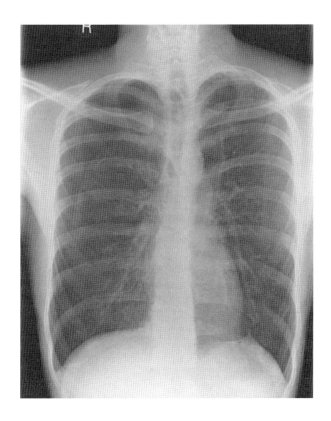

Image quality: _____

Airway: _____

Breathing: _____

Circulation: _____

Diaphragm: _____

Everything else: _____

Diagnosis: _____

Chest X-ray question 7:

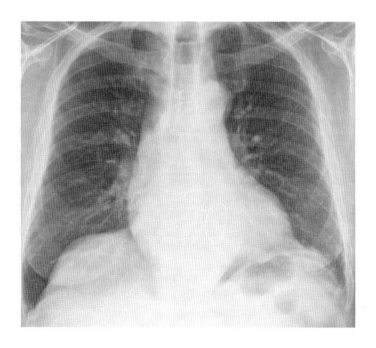

Image quality: _____

Airway: _____

Breathing: _____

Circulation: _____

Diaphragm: _____

Everything else: _____

Diagnosis: _____

Chapter 6

ECG
QUESTIONS

Interpretation questions

Please interpret the following ECGs shown overleaf:

ECG 1

ECG 2

ECG 3

ECG 4

ECG 5

ECG 6

ECG 7

ECG 8

ECG 9

ECG 10

ECQ question 1:

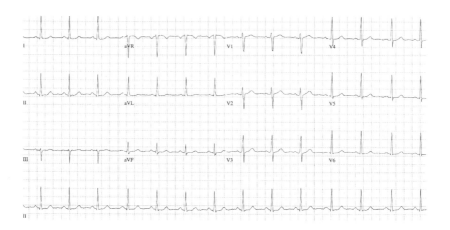

Heart rate: _____

Rhythm: _____

Cardiac axis: _____

P wave morphology: _____

PR interval: _____

QRS complex morphology: _____

ST segment: _____

T wave morphology: _____

Overall: _____

ECG question 2:

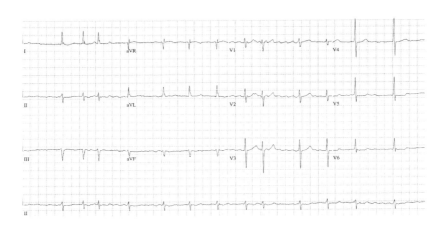

Heart rate: _____

Rhythm: _____

Cardiac axis: _____

P wave morphology: _____

PR interval: _____

QRS complex morphology: _____

ST segment: _____

T wave morphology: _____

Overall: _____

ECG question 3:

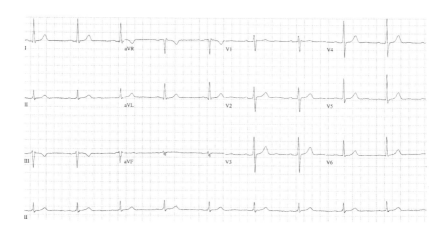

Heart rate: _____

Rhythm: _____

Cardiac axis: _____

P wave morphology: _____

PR interval: _____

QRS complex morphology: _____

ST segment: _____

T wave morphology: _____

Overall: _____

ECG question 4:

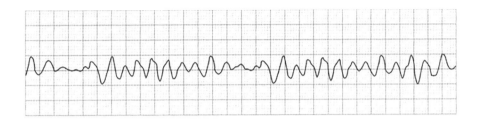

Heart rate: _____

Rhythm: _____

Cardiac axis: _____

P wave morphology: _____

PR interval: _____

QRS complex morphology: _____

ST segment: _____

T wave morphology: _____

Overall: _____

ECG question 5:

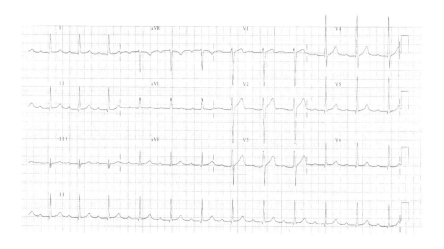

Heart rate: _____

Rhythm: _____

Cardiac axis: _____

P wave morphology: _____

PR interval: _____

QRS complex morphology: _____

ST segment: _____

T wave morphology: _____

Overall: _____

ECG question 6:

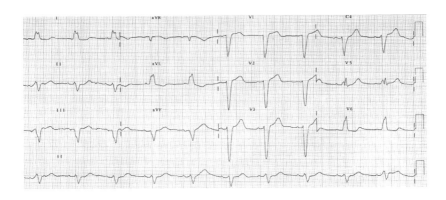

Heart rate: _____

Rhythm: _____

Cardiac axis: _____

P wave morphology: _____

PR interval: _____

QRS complex morphology: _____

ST segment: _____

T wave morphology: _____

Overall: _____

ECQ question 7:

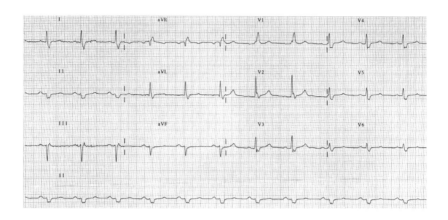

Heart rate: _____

Rhythm: _____

Cardiac axis: _____

P wave morphology: _____

PR interval: _____

QRS complex morphology: _____

ST segment: _____

T wave morphology: _____

Overall: _____

ECG question 8:

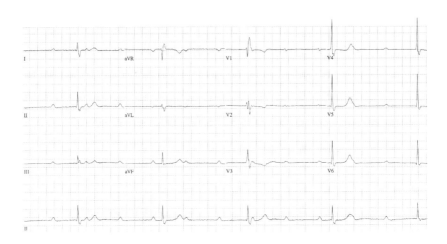

Heart rate: _____

Rhythm: _____

Cardiac axis: _____

P wave morphology: _____

PR interval: _____

QRS complex morphology: _____

ST segment: _____

T wave morphology: _____

Overall: _____

ECG question 9:

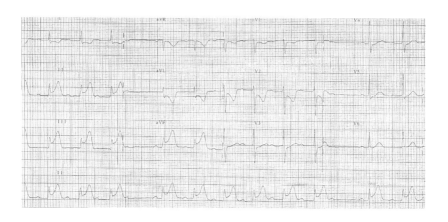

Heart rate: _____

Rhythm: _____

Cardiac axis: _____

P wave morphology: _____

PR interval: _____

QRS complex morphology: _____

ST segment: _____

T wave morphology: _____

Overall: _____

ECG question 10:

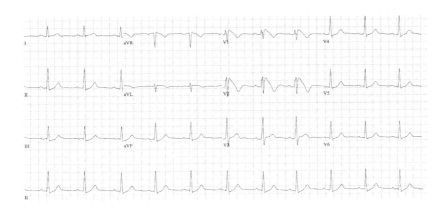

Heart rate: _____

Rhythm: _____

Cardiac axis: _____

P wave morphology: _____

PR interval: _____

QRS complex morphology: _____

ST segment: _____

T wave morphology: _____

Overall: _____

Section 2
Answers

Chapter 7

Practice paper 1
ANSWERS

Single best answers

1) b.
2) a.
3) c.
4) a.
5) b.
6) c.
7) b.
8) d.
9) c.
10) c.
11) b.
12) c.
13) d.
14) d.
15) d.
16) a.
17) a.
18) a.
19) b.
20) c.

21) c.
22) d.
23) c.
24) b.
25) b.
26) d.
27) b.
28) c.
29) a.
30) a.
31) b.
32) c.
33) c.
34) a.
35) a.
36) d.
37) c.
38) d.
39) a.
40) b.

Chapter 8

Practice paper 2
ANSWERS

Extended matching question answers

1) b

   Common features of Williams syndrome include specific facial features including a wide mouth, small upturned nose, teeth and full lips. They have learning disorders, attention deficit hyperactivity disorder, a short stature and speech delays. It is caused by a deletion of genes on chromosome 7.

2) c

   It is important to be aware that a bicuspid aortic valve is the most common cause for aortic stenosis.

3) d

   A ventricular septal defect is a deficiency in the wall separating the left and right ventricles creating a common ventricle. It is associated with a pansystolic murmur along the left sternal border. Larger VSDs may cause a parasternal heave. Smaller defects are associated with a louder murmur. In large defects it is possible for Eisenmenger's syndrome to occur in which the increased pressures in the pulmonary vasculature cause a reversal of a left to right shunt to cause cyanosis.

4) g

Dextrocardia is a rare congenital condition in which the apex of the heart is located on the right side of the body rather than the left. It can be found in isolation or be part of a condition known as situs inversus in which all organs are mirrored.

5) e

An atrial septal defect is a deficit in the wall connecting the atria. There are several different types of atrial septal defects including a patent foramen ovale, ostium secundum, ostium primum, and depend on the area of the atria that is affected. Complications from an ASD include decompression sickness, Eisenmenger's syndrome and paradoxical embolus. ASDs are associated with Down syndrome, fetal alcohol syndrome and Ebstein's anomaly.

6) c

Jaundice, ascites and bruising are features of advanced liver cirrhosis (suggesting portal hypertension and failure of synthetic liver function), thereby making liver failure the most likely cause of the pleural effusion.

7) e

Weight loss, night sweats and lymphadenopathy are suggestive of lymphoma.

8) h

Weight loss and night sweats in a homeless patient who is an ex-IVDU is highly suspicious of tuberculosis. In the immunosuppressed (especially in HIV-positive patients), tuberculosis is more likely to present atypically.

9) f

Worsening oliguria makes renal failure more likely than congestive cardiac failure in this patient with florid fluid overload.

10) b

Dry skin, weight gain and fatigue are typical in hypothyroidism. A macrocytic anaemia can occur. Hypothyroidism can eventually lead to heart failure and fluid retention, resulting in bilateral pleural effusions.

11) f

Bacillus cereus is a Gram-positive bacillus typically infecting contaminated rice and produces two toxins leading to vomiting or diarrhoea. Vomiting usually occurs 2-5 hours after ingestion and diarrhoea 12 hours after ingestion. It usually lasts for 12-24 hours.

12) e

The use of broad-spectrum antibiotics leads to a disruption in the normal bowel flora leading to an overgrowth of *Clostridium difficile* resulting in diarrhoea and possibly pseudomembranous colitis. Treatment is to stop the causative antibiotics, fluid support, oral vancomycin and metronidazole.

13) a

Staphylococcus aureus leads to a rapid onset of symptoms due to the presence of a pre-formed toxin. Symptoms are usually self-limiting and occur following ingestion of contaminated food. Treatment is supportive using fluid management.

14) d

The classical description of symptoms for *Vibrio cholerae* are described in this question; it is transmitted in a faecal-oral route and there is a spectrum of symptoms from mild diarrhoea to severe dehydration. The classical description of the stool appearance is rice water.

15) h

Norovirus is also known as the winter vomiting bug often affecting hospitals or nursing homes. It is transmitted by a faecal-oral route. Symptoms include nausea, vomiting, watery diarrhoea, fever and headaches. Treatment is supportive using fluid management.

16) d

Renal cell carcinoma originates in the cells of the proximal convoluted tubule. It is the most common form of renal cancer in adults accounting for 95% of cases. The classic symptoms are haematuria, flank pain and an abdominal mass on palpation. Risk factors include smoking, obesity, polycyclic aromatic hydrocarbons and asbestos. It is staged using the TNM system.

17) c

Traumatic catheterisation or injury to the urethra due to the pulling on a catheter will lead to epithelial damage and haematuria.

18) d

Renal cell carcinoma originates in the cells of the proximal convoluted tubule. It is the most common form of renal cancer in adults accounting for 95% of cases. The classic symptoms are haematuria, flank pain and an abdominal mass on palpation. Risk factors include smoking, obesity, polycyclic aromatic hydrocarbons and asbestos. It is staged using the TNM system.

19) b

Nephritic syndrome is the presence of haematuria, oliguria, hypertension and glomerulonephritis.

20) h

Common symptoms for bladder cancer includes dysuria, haematuria and lower back pain. The most common type of tumour is a transitional cell carcinoma. Risk factors include smoking, exposure to azo dyes and beta naphthylamine. Superficial tumours can be removed using electrocautery during cystoscopy whilst more invasive tumours can be treated with cystectomy. Immunotherapy using Bacillus Calmette-Guérin (BCG) is used for superficial tumour recurrence.

21) a

Type 1 diabetes has a strong autoimmune link. The antibodies most often associated with this condition are anti-GAD and islet cell antibodies. These contribute to pancreatic islet cell destruction, which is where insulin is produced, and thus the pathological process. HbA1c is a useful test for long-term glucose control.

22) c

These symptoms are of hyperthyroidism, the most common cause of which is Graves' disease. The investigation of choice for this underlying cause is TSH receptor antibodies. Anti-thyroid peroxidase is most associated with Hashimoto's thyroiditis, causing hypothyroidism.

23) d

Hashimoto's disease is often caused by an antibody to thyroid peroxidase.

24) b

Cushing's syndrome is a disease of excess cortisol. This can be from either an endogenous or exogenous source. Some of these endogenous causes are dependent on ACTH. To differentiate between causes, a high-dose dexamethasone suppression test can be used. In a normal test, cortisol should be suppressed by high-dose dexamethasone. If this suppression fails, there is an abnormal excess of cortisol.

25) h

These symptoms are of acromegaly, an excess of growth hormone. The diagnostic test for this is an oral glucose tolerance test. In a normal individual, oral glucose should suppress release and levels of growth hormone. In acromegaly, there is no suppression, and levels may paradoxically rise in response to glucose.

26) e

This is most likely a vascular dementia, which is typified by a stepwise progression. There are multiple vascular risk factors in the history.

27) c

Distressing visual hallucinations and fluctuating cognition are both typical of dementia with Lewy bodies.

28) g

Apathy, personality change and loss of inhibition are all suggestive of frontotemporal dementia.

29) d

A broad-based gait, incontinence and dementia are the core features of normal pressure hydrocephalus.

30) a

The gradual history is consistent with Alzheimer's disease, for which hypercholesterolaemia and diabetes are risk factors.

31) a

Adult haemoglobin is composed of two alpha and two beta chains.

32) e

Alpha thalassaemia minor is a result of a deletion of one of the alpha globulin genes. This is still compatible with life.

33) b

Haemoglobin S is present in sickle cell disease. 'Sickling' of red cells can result in a sickle cell crisis and vaso-occlusive episodes.

34) c

Fetal haemoglobin consists of two alpha and two gamma subunits. Fetal haemoglobin is replaced in the first months of life with adult haemoglobin.

35) h

Adult haemoglobin has a reduced affinity for oxygen compared with fetal haemoglobin. This is necessary, so that fetal haemoglobin can acquire oxygen from adult haemoglobin.

36) d

Cutaneous larva migrans is caused by hookworm larva entering through the skin, most commonly the feet, to cause an intensely itchy rash along the site of the serpiginous track. Walking barefoot on the beach is a risk factor for cutaneous larva migrans.

37) c

There are two clinical subtypes of leishmaniasis, cutaneous and visceral; both are spread by infected sandfly bites. Cutaneous disease presents with a nodule 1-2 months following the bite which ulcerates and crusts over. Visceral leishmaniasis presents with a chronic, progressive history of non-specific symptoms including fever, night sweats, dry cough and nosebleeds. You may find hepatosplenomegaly and lymphadenopathy on examination.

38) a

Schistosomiasis has many different presentations depending on the organism. *Schistosoma haematobium* causes urinary schistosomiasis as in this case and is transmitted in infested water. This can be obtained by drinking or other activities such as swimming.

39) b

African trypanosomiasis is also known as African sleeping sickness and presents with two stages: the first stage with a chancre and non-specific symptoms; the second stage with somnolence and behavioural changes which can progress to a coma.

40) e

Loa loa is also known as the eye worm. It commonly localises to the eye and can be seen moving across the conjunctiva.

41) e

Atlanto-axial instability may present with neck pain. Neurological symptoms from cord or nerve root compression may occur late.

42) f

Upper cranial nerve palsies can complicate giant cell arteritis.

43) d

Mononeuritis multiplex (damage of two or more peripheral nerves in differing locations) are seen in PAN as a result of ischaemic nerve damage from vasculitis.

44) c

Carpal tunnel syndrome is common in rheumatoid arthritis.

45) h

Psychiatric symptoms associated with the use of steroids are very common and can occur at any time during treatment.

46) d

Multiple endocrine neoplasia Type 1 is the presence of medullary thyroid carcinoma, phaeochromocytoma in addition to mucosal neuromas and a marfanoid body habitus. It is caused by a mutation in the RET proto-oncogene on chromosome 10.

47) f

Multiple endocrine neoplasia Type 2B is the presence of a pituitary tumour, parathyroid hyperplasia and pancreatic tumours. It is caused by a mutation in the MEN1 gene.

48) b

Pancreatic cancer is the fifth most common cancer in the UK. It is characterised by epigastric pain radiating to the back, painless jaundice and features of malabsorption. Thrombophlebitis migrans is the transient swelling and redness of different limb veins due to clot formation. It is important to remember Courvoisier's law in relation to painless jaundice; this states that in the presence of a palpable gallbladder painless jaundice is unlikely to be due to gallstones. This holds true as the formation of gallstones results in a fibrotic shrunken gallbladder that does not easily distend.

49) g

These are rare biliary tree tumours associated with conditions such as primary sclerosing cholangitis or inflammatory bowel disease. Symptoms include obstructive jaundice, weight loss, steatorrhoea and epigastric pain.

50) h

Gallbladder tumours are rare and may be found incidentally during a cholecystectomy; however, some patients present with symptoms such as right upper quadrant pain, vomiting and nausea with weight loss and obstructive jaundice. CA-19 and CEA may be raised.

51) f

This patient probably has steroid-induced pancreatitis. Serum amylase is most useful in the acute setting; urinary amylase can be used if presentation is delayed as it remains elevated for longer.

52) d

This patient most probably has diverticulitis and a CT scan is most appropriate to diagnose this and assess for complications.

53) a

This patient does not present with enough signs of appendicitis to do an emergency laparoscopy straight away. An ultrasound can diagnose appendicitis or other causes such as gynaecological pathology.

54) b

This patient probably has a postoperative ileus. An X-ray will show dilated bowel loops and is easily and quickly performed.

55) h

This patient has a postoperative wound infection. A wound swab will show the responsible organism and antibiotic sensitivities, so the appropriate antibiotics can be given.

56) a

This patient has a fibroadenoma which are relatively common in this age group with a peak incidence at 20 years. They arise from the entire lobule with both stromal and epithelial components. There is no increased risk of malignancy. They are often referred to as 'breast mice' due to their discrete, firm and mobile nature.

57) f

This patient has a seroma. These do not tend to collect immediately after surgery so people notice them over the coming weeks. This mastectomy with axillary node clearance provides a potential space for fluid to accumulate. Unlike an abscess or cellulitis, patients are usually well, and symptoms relate to size and pressure on surrounding structures.

58) e

Lipomas are common and can occur anywhere on the body. This patient is young and the lump is described as superficial. There are no worrying features in the history; if there were any concerns, a referral to dermatology/breast services would be appropriate.

59) d

Ductal carcinoma *in situ* is the most common type of breast cancer and is a malignancy of the ductal breast tissue but with an intact basement membrane. 20-30% of cases develop invasive disease. It is often detected by screening which shows macrocalcification tracking along the duct. The treatment is by a wide local excision or mastectomy.

60) b

This patient most likely has an area of fat necrosis due to trauma from her seatbelt. She would still need to be assessed in the breast clinic using a triple assessment which includes a full history and examination, and a radiological and histological examination to rule out other breast pathology.

61) b

Tamsulosin would be the first-line treatment but this causes hypotension as it is an alpha blocker, so finasteride is more appropriate in this instance.

62) e

Patients with suspected prostate malignancy should undergo an MRI to guide decision making about biopsy and treatment.

63) c

Patients with LUTS caused by benign prostatic enlargement refractory to pharmacological treatment may be offered surgical treatment, most commonly TURP.

64) h

This patient has locally advanced malignant disease and a poor performance status so no curative treatments are available. Radiotherapy may be effective for managing bone metastases.

65) f

These investigation findings suggest malignancy. As the anterior prostate is not accessible via the transrectal approach, a perineal approach will be more appropriate.

66) f

This patient scores 9. E — opens eyes to voice (3), V — incomprehensible sounds (2), M — withdraws to pain (4).

67) d

This patient scores 15. E — opens eyes spontaneously (4), V — orientated (5), M — obeys commands (6).

68) g

This patient scores 3. E — no response (1), V — no response (1), M — no response (1).

69) h

This patient scores 10. E — opens eyes to pain (2), V — confused (4), M — withdraws to pain (4).

70) e

This patient scores 12. E — opens eyes to voice (3), V — inappropriate words (3), M — obeys commands (6).

71) a

Stanford Type B dissections involve the descending aorta distal to the left subclavian artery. They are treated with medical therapy through control of hypertension.

72) e

Acute limb ischaemia is a surgical emergency and requires treatment within 6 hours of symptom onset to preserve the limb. Embolism accounts for 30% of cases of acute lower limb ischaemia.

73) b

Varicose veins can be treated with reassurance and graduated compression stockings for first-line medical therapy.

74) a

The first-line management for intermittent claudication is to encourage a healthy diet, weight loss, control of comorbidities and risk factors such as hypertension, diabetes, cholesterol and smoking.

75) c

If patients opt for surgical management of varicose veins, then several approaches can be considered including ligation with stripping, sclerotherapy or endovenous laser ablation. Sclerotherapy is not recommended for patients using the oral contraceptive pill or hormone replacement therapy.

76) f

A Monteggia fracture is a fracture of the proximal third of the ulna with dislocation of the proximal radial head. It usually requires surgery.

77) a

A Colles' fracture is a common fracture of frailty. It should be reduced promptly and stabilised in a cast. If there is a good reduction, and radial height and inclination are maintained, it may be treated non-operatively.

78) e

A Galeazzi fracture is a fracture of the distal third of the radius with dislocation of the distal radioulnar joint. It usually requires surgery.

79) c

A Bennett's fracture can be treated non-operatively if there is a good reduction in a cast but the likelihood of a stiff thumb is high, so patient factors are important in the decision-making process.

80) h

A boxer's fracture is often treated non-operatively if there is no rotational deformity (i.e. do all the fingers point to the thenar eminence when they make a fist).

81) e

The normal pH is 7.35-7.45.

82) a

The normal PaO_2 is 11-13kPa.

83) c

The normal bicarbonate is 22-28mmol/L.

84) f

The normal base excess is -2 to +2 and is the amount of acid or alkali to restore 1L of oxygenated blood to a normal pH at a $PaCO_2$ of 5.3kPa at 37°C.

85) h

The normal anion gap is 12-16 and is calculated by $Na^+ + K^+ - (Cl^- + HCO_3^-)$.

86) c

In a child, parotid swelling is much more likely to be caused by infection than a tumour. Mumps may occur in vaccinated children.

87) h

Carbamazepine is a licensed treatment for trigeminal neuralgia.

88) d

Exposure to wood dust is a risk factor for nasopharyngeal carcinoma. The history of exposure and the unilateral nasal blockage should make malignancy a concern in this patient.

89) a

Although the presentation is similar to the previous patient, the shorter history and bilateral nasal blockage suggest a benign cause is more likely.

90) a

The history is suggestive of acute sinusitis involving the frontal sinus.

91) e

This patient should have a bowel resection performed; this could be a potentially curative treatment.

92) a

Head and neck tumours are often treated with combined chemotherapy or radiotherapy. HPV-related tumours have a very high cure rate using this treatment.

93) b

Small cell lung cancer can be very aggressive but also very sensitive to chemotherapy. It responds poorly to radiotherapy and given the location (close to mediastinum) radiotherapy would not be indicated.

94) g

A Whipple's procedure is a potentially curative surgery for pancreatic cancer. Pancreatic cancer has a very poor prognosis and high mortality rate.

95) b

Germ cell testicular cancers are highly responsive to chemotherapy; even metastatic germ cell tumours can be cured with chemotherapy.

96) d

Pregnancy can cause a rapid progression of diabetic retinopathy; good diabetic control can help prevent deterioration. Proliferative retinopathy is the presence of new vessel growth within the retina.

97) h

Hypertensive retinopathy is retinal damage due to high blood pressure. This patient has a Grade 2 hypertensive retinopathy which is characterised by arteriole constriction and areas of focal irregularities. The presence of retinal haemorrhages or exudates are Grade 3 and the presence of disc swelling alongside all other signs is Grade 4.

98) e

Age-related macular degeneration (ARMD) results in the blurring or loss of central vision and is the result of damage to the macula. It is thought that drusen deposits within Bruch's membrane which separates retinal pigment epithelium and the retina from the underlying choroidal blood supply, leading to disruption of nutrient delivery and removal causing retinal atrophy. If a break in Bruch's membrane occurs, fragile blood vessels can grow directly into the retina and if these are damaged, haemorrhage and oedema occur resulting in loss of central vision. There are two types of ARMD — wet and dry. The dry type is the presence of drusen and retinal pigment epithelial atrophy whilst the wet type is the neovascularisation of the retina and subsequent bleeding.

99) h

A sudden loss of vision in a known hypertensive patient should prompt a clinician to immediately consider an underlying vascular cause. The central retinal vein drains all retinal layers and optic nerve; when occluded there is venous engorgement, retinal oedema, ischaemia and haemorrhage. It is one of the most common causes of sudden unilateral vision loss. It is associated with diabetes and hypertension.

100) c

Retinopathy of prematurity occurs in low weight or pre-term babies and is associated with a use of high oxygen concentrations in neonatal life; however, other factors such as sepsis and blood transfusion have been thought to drive this pathology. Fundoscopy will reveal a ridge of tissue with blood vessel growth to that area. It can resolve or progress leading to contraction and detachment of the retina. Treatments include laser ablation to the affected area.

101) c

Lithium toxicity presents with a wide variety of symptoms including ataxia, coarse tremor and dysarthria. A fine tremor is a common side effect of lithium therapy that is not indicative of toxicity.

102) b

Aspirin overdose presents with gastrointestinal symptoms and ringing in the ears. Patients classically hyperventilate due to stimulation of the respiratory centre leading to respiratory alkalosis.

103) f

Flumazenil can be used to reverse an overdose of benzodiazepines. This is rarely used as it reduces the seizure threshold.

104) g

An opiate overdose presents with a reduced respiratory rate, 'pinpoint' pupils and a reduced GCS. Naloxone is used for the reversal of an opiate overdose; this is short-acting in comparison to the effects of opiates, therefore, it may need to be repeated.

105) e

Paracetamol overdose (intentional or unintentional) is the most common cause of acute liver failure in the United Kingdom. It is treated with intravenous N-acetylcysteine.

106) a

The 6-in-1 vaccine, protecting against diphtheria, tetanus, whooping cough, polio, *Haemophilus influenzae* type B and hepatitis B.

107) g

Protects against measles, mumps and rubella.

108) h

The 3-in-1 vaccine protects against tetanus, diphtheria and polio.

109) d

Protects against rotavirus infection.

110) e

Protects against the human papilloma virus.

111) h

This bacteria causes the sexually transmitted infection, syphilis, which initially presents as a painless chancre and its prevalence is increasing in older adults.

112) f

A common sexually transmitted infection which appears as a Gram-negative diplococcus.

113) g

Clue cells are characteristic of bacterial vaginosis and *Gardnerella* is the most common causative organism of this infection.

114) d

Painful ulcers are synonymous with herpes unless proven otherwise as there are other non-infective causes of this lesion.

115) c

This is a protozoal sexually transmitted infection which is also increasing in prevalence.

116) a

Neurofibromatosis is a condition characterised by tumour growth in the nervous system. This case is suggestive of neurofibromatosis Type 1. The light-brown flat macules are also known as cafe-au-lait spots.

117) e

The long-term administration of amiodarone is associated with blue-grey discolouration. It is a useful anti-arrhythmic drug; however, it has a lot of side effects including interstitial lung disease, thyroid abnormalities and deranged liver function tests.

118) f

Addison's disease is primary adrenal sufficiency most commonly due to autoimmune disease. Presentation can be vague with non-specific symptoms such as fatigue, anorexia and abdominal pain. Hyperpigmentation may be found on examination, particularly of the buccal mucosa, skin folds and pressure areas.

119) h

Tuberous sclerosis is characterised by the development of hamartomas in many different systems. It may present with infantile spasms in infancy and ash leaf macules are characteristic; a Wood's lamp can be used to visualise these more easily.

120) c

Vitiligo is destruction of the melanocytes. It presents with discrete white patches of skin and is associated with autoimmune disease.

121) h

PPIs inhibit H^+/K^+ ATPase to reduce acid secretion in the stomach.

122) f

Salbutamol is a beta-2 agonist that acts to cause airway smooth muscle cells to relax. It can cause a tachycardia and reduce serum potassium levels. The inhaler form usually has an onset of 15 minutes and lasts for up to 6 hours.

123) d

Clopidogrel is an antiplatelet medication that is used to reduce the risk of myocardial infarction and stroke in patients that are at a higher risk of these events. It can also be used in the treatment of MI and during coronary artery stent insertion.

124) c

Aspirin is a non-selective COX inhibitor and irreversibly binds to platelets. It blocks the formation of thromboxane A2 to prevent platelet aggregation for the life of the affected platelet which is usually 8-9 days.

125) a

Warfarin is a vitamin K antagonist which acts to inhibit the formation of vitamin K-dependent clotting factors II, VII, IX and X. The effect of warfarin is measured using the International Normalised Ratio (INR).

126) a

Co-amoxiclav is a beta-lactam antibiotic that inhibits cell wall synthesis. It is formed from amoxicillin and potassium clavulanate and is commonly used for otitis media, pneumonia, UTI and cellulitis.

127) h

Erythromycin is a macrolide antibiotic that works by inhibiting protein synthesis of the 50S subunit. It is often used in those who are allergic to penicillin and it is active against *Streptococcus*, *Staphylococcus*, *Haemophilus* and *Corynebacterium*.

128) f

Gentamicin is an aminoglycoside that inhibits the 30S subunit to inhibit protein synthesis. It is used in the treatment of osteomyelitis, endocarditis, pelvic inflammatory disease, pneumonia and UTI. Side effects include ototoxicity and nephrotoxicity.

129) g

Trimethoprim acts to inhibit folic acid synthesis to prevent the formation of purines which can be utilised to make bacterial DNA.

130) e

Vancomycin acts to inhibit bacterial cell wall synthesis and is typically used in the treatment of *C. difficile*-related diarrhoea. It is given in the oral form for this condition to ensure effectiveness.

131) a

Sensitivity is the ability of a test to identify a patient with a disease as a positive result.

132) b

Specificity is the ability of a test to identify a patient without the disease as a negative result.

133) d

A positive predicted value is the probability that a patient with a positive test result actually has the disease.

134) e

A negative predicted value is the probability that a patient with a negative test result does not have the disease.

135) h

The prevalence of a condition is the proportion of a population with a disease within a specific time period.

136) e

Deontology is concerned with the worthiness of an action and involves assessing the duties and rights.

137) g

Consequentialism is concerned with the outcome of a particular behaviour.

138) f

Virtue ethics assesses whether the person acting is performing the action for a positive reason.

139) d

Non-maleficence is the principle of avoiding causing harm.

140) a

Autonomy is concerned with ensuring the patient is able to form their own decision; this contrasts to paternalism in which the decision is often made without their input; for example, a doctor making a treatment choice without any patient input.

Chapter 9

Practice paper 3
ANSWERS

Short answer question answers

1)
a. Coronary vasodilation.   2 marks
   Reducing heart rate.
b. Coronary angiogram.   1 mark
c. Antiplatelets.   4 marks
   Statins.
   Antihypertensives.
   Angiotensin-converting enzyme inhibitors.
d. Coronary artery bypass graft.   1 mark
e. Any 2 from: 2 marks
   - Cerebrovascular accident.
   - Myocardial infarction.
   - Pericardial tamponade.
   - Haemothorax.
   - Post-perfusion syndrome.
   - Postoperative atrial fibrillation.
   - Wound site infection.
   - Stenosis.
   - Non-union of sternum.

2)

a.   Chest drain.   1 mark

b.   Any 3 from: 3 marks
   ● Ehlers-Danlos syndrome.
   ● Marfan syndrome.
   ● Pulmonary fibrosis.
   ● Sarcoidosis.
   ● COPD.

c.   Any 3 from: 3 marks
   ● Raised JVP.
   ● Trachea displaced away from the side of the pneumothorax.
   ● Raised heart rate.
   ● Reduced blood pressure.

d.   The British Thoracic Society suggests a measurement from the chest   1 mark
   wall to the outer edge of the lung at the level of the hilum.

e.   Any 2 from: 2 marks
   ● Surgical pleurodesis.
   ● Thoracotomy and pleurectomy.
   ● Video-assisted thoracoscopy.

3)

a.   Oesophageal carcinoma.   1 mark

b.   Any 4 from: 2 marks
   ● Smoking.
   ● Increasing age.
   ● Low-fibre diet.
   ● Alcohol.
   ● Hot beverages.
   ● Achalasia.
   ● Tylosis.
   ● Plummer-Vinson syndrome.
   ● Thoracic radiotherapy.
   ● GORD.

- Barrett's oesophagus.
- Obesity.
- Male sex.
- Diet high in pickled foods.

c. Any 3 from: 3 marks
- Pharyngeal pouch.
- Pharyngeal carcinoma.
- Oesophageal web.
- Foreign body.
- Stroke.
- Oesophagitis.
- Oesophageal stricture.
- Achalasia.
- Oesophageal spasm.
- Bulbar palsy.
- Myasthenia gravis.
- Multiple sclerosis.
- Parkinson's disease.
- External compression from lung cancer.
- Retrosternal thyroid.

d. Any 2 from: 2 marks
- Barium swallow.
- Routine bloods.
- Chest X-ray.
- CT scan.
- OGD.
- PET scan.

e. Any 2 from: 2 marks
- Multidisciplinary team (MDT) meeting.
- Radiofrequency ablation.
- Stenting.
- Endoscopic mucosal resection.
- Neoadjuvant chemotherapy.

- Oesophagostomy.
- Palliative support.
- Dietician review.

4)

a. Urinary outflow obstruction (1 mark); for example, blockage of a catheter, calculi, enlarged prostate (1 mark). 2 marks

b. Any 2 from: 2 marks
   - Bladder scan.
   - Flush catheter.
   - Change of catheter.

c. Any 3 from: 3 marks
   - White cell count.
   - Neutrophils.
   - CRP.
   - Alkaline phosphatase.
   - Ferritin.

d. Any 2 from: 2 marks
   - Previous pelvic cancers.
   - Previous lower abdominal or pelvic surgery.
   - Coagulopathy.

e. NSAIDs, e.g. ibuprofen, naproxen or aspirin. 1 mark

5)

a. Beta (1 mark) pancreatic islet cells (1 mark). 2 marks

b. Any 1 from: 2 marks
   - HLA-DR3.
   - HLA-DR4.

c. Any 1 from: 1 mark
   - Anti-GAD.
   - Islet cell antibodies.

d. >11.0mmol/L. 2 marks

e.   Any 3 from: 3 marks
   ● DKA.
   ● Retinopathy.
   ● Nephropathy.
   ● Neuropathy.
   ● PVD.
   ● CVD.
   ● Postural hypotension.

6)
a.   Any 2 from: 2 marks
   ● Antibody-mediated inflammation.
   ● Demyelinating plaques.
   ● Slowed neurotransmission.
b.   Uhthoff's phenomenon.   1 mark
c.   Any 2 from: 4 marks
   ● Reduced visual evoked potentials.
   ● High T2-signal intensity lesions on MRI.
   ● Oligoclonal bands on CSF electrophoresis.
d.   Corticosteroids.   1 mark
e.   Any 2 from: 2 marks
   ● Beta-interferon.
   ● Glatiramer acetate.
   ● Natalizumab.
   ● Fingolimod.
   ● Mitoxantrone.
   ● Azathioprine.
   ● Teriflunomide.
   ● Alemtuzumab.
   ● Dimethyl fumarate.

7)
a.   Fibrin strands are deposited in vessels and 'chop-up' red cells.   1 mark
b.   Any 3 from: 3 marks
  - Diarrhoea.
  - Renal failure.
  - Itching.
  - Anuria.
  - Oedema.
  - Fever.
c.   Neurological system.   2 marks
d.   Helmet cells.   2 marks
      Schistocytes.
e.   Von Willebrand factor cleaving protease.   2 marks

8)
a.   Any 3 from: 3 marks
  - Rhinovirus.
  - Coronavirus.
  - Adenovirus.
  - Respiratory syncytial virus.
  - Parainfluenza virus.
  - Metapneumovirus.
b.   Haemagglutinin.   2 marks
      Neuraminidase.
c.   Antigenic shift.   1 mark
d.   Any 6 from: 3 marks
  - Cholera.
  - Dengue fever.
  - Diphtheria.
  - *Haemophilus influenzae* type B.
  - Hepatitis A.
  - Hepatitis B.
  - Hepatitis E.

- Human papilloma virus.
- Japanese encephalitis.
- Malaria.
- Measles.
- Meningococcal disease.
- Mumps.
- Pertussis.
- Pneumococcal disease.
- Polio.
- Rabies.
- Rotavirus.
- Rubella.
- Tetanus.
- Tick-borne encephalitis.
- Tuberculosis.
- Typhoid fever.
- Varicella zoster.
- Yellow fever.

e. Any 1 from: 1 mark
    - Oseltamivir (Tamiflu®).
    - Zanamivir.

9)

a. Anti-centromere.   2 marks
    Anti-Scl 70/anti-topoisomerase.

b. Any 3 from: 3 marks
    - Microstomia.
    - Telangiectasia.
    - Calcinosis.
    - Sclerodactyly.
    - Hypopigmentation.
    - Hyperpigmentation.
    - Fingertip lesions.
    - Abnormal nailfold capillaries.

c.   Pulmonary fibrosis.   2 marks
      Pulmonary hypertension.
d.   Calcium channel blocker.   2 marks
      Nifedipine.
e.   PPI therapy.   1 mark

10)
a.   Any 4 from: 2 marks
- Acute cholecystitis.
- Ascending cholangitis.
- Biliary colic.
- Hepatitis.
- Hepatic abscess.
- Empyema of the gallbladder.
- Colonic tumour of hepatic flexure.
- Pneumonia.
- Pulmonary embolism.
- Peptic ulcer.
- Gastritis.
- Duodenitis.
- Intestinal obstruction.
- Pancreatitis.
- Inflammatory bowel disease.
- Retrocaecal appendicitis.
- Pyelonephritis.
- Renal stones.
- Herpes zoster.
- Myocardial infarction.
- Pericarditis.

b.   Any 4 from: 2 marks
- Full blood count.
- Urea & Electrolytes.
- Liver function tests.

- Clotting.
- CRP.
- Amylase.
- Chest X-ray.
- Urinalysis.
- Abdominal X-ray.
- Ultrasound.
- CT.
- ECG.

c. Acute cholecystitis.   1 mark

d. Any 2 from: 2 marks
  - Analgesia.
  - Antibiotics.
  - IV fluids.
  - Vitamin K.
  - Antiemetics.
  - Laparoscopic cholecystectomy.

e. Any 3 from: 3 marks
  - Ascending cholangitis.
  - Empyema.
  - Gallstone ileus.
  - Pancreatitis.
  - Chronic cholecystitis.
  - Common bile duct stone.
  - Gallbladder rupture.

11)

a. Any 2 from: 2 marks
  - Abdominal tenderness.
  - Peritonism.
  - Faeculent or purulent material in the surgical drain.
  - Pyrexia.
  - Tachycardia.

b.   CT abdomen.   1 mark

c.   Any 2 from: 2 marks
  - Peritoneal contamination.
  - Obesity.
  - Diabetes.
  - Immunosuppression.
  - Emergency surgery.
  - Smoking.
  - Excessive alcohol.
  - Oesophageal/rectal anastomosis.

d.   Any 3 from: 3 marks
  - Wound infection.
  - Intra-abdominal collection.
  - Incontinence.
  - Bleeding.
  - Obstruction.
  - Incisional hernia.

e.   If there is a minor leak on CT it can be treated conservatively with   2 marks
       bowel rest and antibiotics. A drain may also be needed (1 mark). A
       major leak needs a laparotomy and washout with repair (1 mark).

12)

a.   The patient can understand the information given to them (0.5 mark),   2 marks
       retain it (0.5 mark), weigh up the information (0.5 mark) and
       communicate their decision back to you (0.5 mark).

b.   Offer all patients a chaperone.   1 mark

c.   Inspection (with relaxed and tensed pectoral muscles).   4 marks
       Palpation with systematic approach, e.g. clock face starting with the
       normal breast.
       Examine axillary tail and nipple.
       Examine any lumps individually.

d.   Any 2 from: 2 marks
  - Axillary lymph nodes.
  - Head lymph nodes.

- Neck lymph nodes.
- Inguinal lymph nodes.

e.   The patient should not be sent home without any follow-up. It has   1 mark
      been some time since her last screening and she is over 50. She
      should be referred to the breast clinic for a more thorough
      assessment.

13)

a.   Phimosis is narrowing of the opening of the foreskin (1 mark), often   2 marks
      such that it cannot be retracted fully or at all, whereas paraphimosis
      is a condition in which the retracted foreskin remains stuck behind
      the glans and cannot return to its original position (1 mark).

b.   No, phimosis may be physiological up to the age of 3-5 years.   1 mark

c.   Paraphimosis is a urological emergency (1 mark). Early cases should   3 marks
      be treated by manual compression of the swollen foreskin with
      counter pressure on the glans using a saline-soaked gauze (1 mark).
      Late or severe cases may need surgical reduction, often with a dorsal
      slit or full circumcision (1 mark).

d.   An abnormally sustained erection that is not related to sexual   1 mark
      stimulation. It can be high-flow (arterial) or low-flow (venous
      congestion).

e.   Any 3 from: 3 marks
      - Low-flow: medication adverse effect, e.g. chlorpromazine.
      - Blood disorders affecting viscosity, e.g. sickle cell.
      - Neurological disease, e.g. spinal disease or stroke.
      - High-flow causes: trauma to the penis or perineum.

14)

a.   Glioma.   1 mark

b.   Any 2 from: 2 marks
      - Meningioma.
      - Glioblastoma multiforme.
      - Cerebral lymphoma.

- Medulloblastoma.
- Acoustic neuroma.
- Neurofibroma.
- Pineal tumour.
- Craniopharyngioma.

c. Frontal lobe. 1 mark
d. Chemotherapy. 3 marks
Radiotherapy.
Surgery.
e. Any 3 from: 3 marks
- Aggressive.
- Fast-growing.
- Poorly differentiated.
- High mitotic activity.

15)
a. Intermittent claudication. 1 mark
b. Any 3 from: 3 marks
- Smoking.
- Diabetes.
- Hypercholesterolaemia.
- Hypertension.
- Family history of hyperhomocysteinaemia.
- Cardiovascular disease.

c. Any 2 from: 2 marks
- Smoking cessation.
- Weight loss.
- Regular exercise.
- Good glycaemic control.
- Controlling hypertension.
- Increase exercise tolerance.
- Antiplatelet agents.
- Statin therapy.

d. Any 2 from: 2 marks
    - ECG.
    - ABPI.
    - Duplex Doppler.
    - Arteriography.
    - Magnetic resonance angiogram.

e. Any 2 from: 2 marks
    - Angioplasty.
    - Stenting.
    - Bypass grafting.
    - Amputation.

16)

a. Sciatica is pain arising from anywhere along the path of the sciatic   3 marks
    nerve (1 mark).
    Any 2 from:
    - Intervertebral disc herniation.
    - Spinal stenosis.
    - Spondylolisthesis.
    - Pelvic tumours.
    - Compression from fetal head during pregnancy.

b. Any 4 from: 2 marks
    - Age >55 years.
    - Male.
    - Known malignancy.
    - Bladder/bowel dysfunction.
    - Unexplained weight loss.
    - Intravenous drug use.
    - Immunosuppression.
    - Night sweats.
    - History of trauma.
    - Nocturnal pain.
    - Bilateral sciatica.

  - Peripheral neurological deficit.
  - Saddle anaesthesia.

c.   Cauda equina syndrome describes a condition characterised by lower   2 marks
     back pain radiating down the leg, saddle anaesthesia and
     urinary/faecal disturbance (1 mark).
     The cauda equina portion of the spinal cord (horse's tail) is
     compressed leading to progressive neurological deficit which if left
     untreated can result in loss of sensorimotor function in the lower
     limbs (1 mark).

d.   Any 2 from: 2 marks
  - Age.
  - Description of neuropathic type pain originating in the back.
  - Radiating down the leg.
  - Insensate urinary retention.
  - Sensory loss in the distribution of L5.
  - Loss of motor function and reflexes are a late sign.

e.   Urgent MRI.   1 mark

17)

a.   Colloid.   1 mark

b.   Permissive hypotension is a strategy used in the resuscitation of   2 marks
     bleeding trauma patients. This advocates the cautious use of fluid to
     maintain a blood pressure lower than normal but that can sustain
     sufficient organ perfusion; this is believed to prevent a large increase
     in blood pressure to disrupt clot formation.

c.   Any 4 from: 4 marks
  - Haemolysis.
  - Non-haemolytic febrile reaction.
  - Urticaria.
  - Pruritus.
  - Coagulopathy.
  - Anaphylaxis.
  - Transfusion-related acute lung injury (TRALI).
  - Thrombocytopaenia.

- Transfusion-associated circulatory overload (TACO).
- Sepsis.
- Hyperkalaemia.
- Hypocalcaemia.
- Graft vs. host disease.
- Infectious disease transmission.
- Hypothermia.
- Iron overload.

d. Any 2 from: 1 mark
- Iron overload.
- Hyperkalaemia.
- Hypocalcaemia.

e. Any 2 from: 2 marks
- 0.9% normal saline.
- Hartmann's solution.
- Glucose.
- Gelatin solutions such as Gelofusine®.
- Starch-based fluids such as Voluven®.
- Dextrans.
- Recombinant factor VIIa.
- IV iron.
- Recombinant erythropoietin if free from human albumin.
- Some individuals may consider cell salvage, haemodilution, haemodialysis or cardiac bypass. Hospitals have access to the Hospital Liaison Committee for Jehovah's Witnesses and they can provide support and information should they be required.

18)

a. Ramsay Hunt syndrome is caused by reactivation of a varicella zoster   2 marks
infection (1 mark) in the geniculate ganglion of the facial nerve within
the temporal bone (1 mark). This usually results in a vesicular rash
and acute lower motor neurone facial nerve palsy.

b. Any 2 from: 2 marks
    - Vertigo.
    - Headaches.
    - Dysarthria.
    - Ataxic gait.
    - Fever.
    - Cervical lymphadenopathy.
    - Tinnitus.

c. Acyclovir.   2 marks
    Oral corticosteroids.

d. Any 2 from: 2 marks
    - Vestibular sedatives for vertigo.
    - Analgesia.
    - Carbamazepine for pain.
    - Eyedrops.
    - Taping eye at night if unable to close the eye.

e. Most patients recover well with resolution of symptoms (1 mark).   2 marks
    However, more than half of patients have some degree of permanent
    facial weakness (1 mark).

19)

a. Any 2 from: 2 marks
    - Dysphagia.
    - Vomiting.
    - Weight loss.
    - Anorexia.
    - Weight loss.
    - Melena.

b. Microcytic anaemia.   1 mark

c. Barrett's oesophagus (1 mark) — caused by chronic acid reflux (1   3 marks
    mark). Metaplasia — columnar epithelium (gastric mucosa) extends
    into the lower oesophagus replacing squamous epithelium (1 mark).

d.   Stenting procedure.   2 marks
      Refeeding syndrome.
e.   Recurrent (1 mark) laryngeal nerve palsy (1 mark).   2 marks

20)
a.   Bacterial conjunctivitis.   1 mark
b.   Any 4 from: 2 marks
      ● Episcleritis.
      ● Scleritis.
      ● Corneal foreign body or abrasion.
      ● Ocular trauma.
      ● Acute closed angle glaucoma.
      ● Iritis.
      ● Subconjunctival haemorrhage.
      ● Anterior uveitis.
      ● Corneal ulcer.
      ● Keratitis.
      ● Corneal abscess.
      ● Blepharitis.
      ● Endophthalmitis.
      ● Allergic or viral conjunctivitis.
c.   Any 3 from: 3 marks
      ● Eyelids.
      ● Eyelashes.
      ● Blink reflex.
      ● Tear film.
      ● Intact corneal or conjunctival epithelium provides a mechanical
        barrier.
      ● MALT tissue in conjunctiva.
d.   Viral cause: adenovirus.   3 marks
      Any 2 from bacterial causes:
      ● *Staphylococcus epidermidis*.
      ● *Staphylococcus aureus*.

- *Streptococcus pneumoniae.*
- *Haemophilus influenzae.*
- *Moraxella lacunata.*

e)   Any 1 comparison from Table 9.1 below.   1 mark

Table 9.1

	Bacterial conjunctivitis	Viral conjunctivitis
Discharge	Purulent	Watery
Chemosis	Mild	Moderate
Tarsal conjunctiva	Papillae	Follicles
Pre-auricular lymphadenopathy	Occasional	Common

21)

a.   Any 2 from: 2 marks
- REM sleep disturbance.
- Sensitivity to antipsychotic medication.
- Autonomic dysfunction.
- Hallucinations in other modalities.
- Hypersomnia.
- Apathy.
- Falls.

b.   Tremor.   3 marks
Rigidity.
Bradykinesia.

c. Any 3 from: 3 marks
    - Alzheimer's disease.
    - Vascular dementia.
    - Frontotemporal dementia.
    - Huntington's disease.
    - Normal pressure hydrocephalus.
    - Mixed dementia.
    - Corticobasal degeneration.
    - Progressive supranuclear palsy.
    - HIV infection.
    - Creutzfeldt-Jakob disease.

d. Any 1 from: 1 mark
    - Donepezil
    - Rivastigmine.

e. Progressive supranuclear palsy.   1 mark

22)

a. Abnormal sputum means mucociliary clearance is reduced, resulting   1 mark
    in recurrent infections.

b. Delta F508 gene mutation (1 mark) in the CFTR gene encoding for the 2 marks
    CFTR protein (1 mark).

c. Any 3 from: 3 marks
    - Lungs.
    - Bowels.
    - Pancreas.
    - Liver.
    - Infertility.
    - Bone (osteoporosis).

d. Sweat test (high chloride concentration).   1 mark

e. Any 3 from: 3 marks
    - Mucus clearance to prevent infections.
    - Chest physiotherapy.
    - Physical exercise.

- Bronchodilator therapy.
- Mannitol.
- Organ transplant.
- Pancreatic enzyme replacement.
- Weight advice.
- Insulin.
- Vitamin D.
- Reproductive advice.
- Psychological support.
- Calcium.
- Bisphosphonates.
- Vaccination against influenza and pneumococcus.

23)
a. 1 in 10. 1 mark
b. Any 5 from: 5 marks
  - Pre-existing mental health illness.
  - Family or personal history of postnatal depression.
  - Single parenthood.
  - Social isolation.
  - Emotional stresses in the postpartum period.
c. SSRIs. 2 marks
SNRIs.
d. Postpartum psychosis. 1 mark
e. Bipolar disorder. 1 mark

24)
a. Any 3 from: 3 marks
  - Flushed appearance.
  - Warm or moist skin.
  - Thin hair.
  - Hair loss.
  - Thyroid acropachy.

- Onycholysis.
- Pruritus.
- Urticaria.
- Pretibial myxoedema.
- Palmar erythema.

b.   Any 3 from: 3 marks

- Cold skin.
- Dry or coarse skin.
- Dermatitis.
- Sparse or brittle hair.
- Loss of eyebrow hair.
- Brittle nails.
- Ridges on the nails.
- Myxoedema.

c.   Graves' disease.   2 marks

d.   Any 1 from: 1 mark

- Carbimazole.
- Propylthiouracil.

e.   Thyroid storm.   1 mark

25)

Table 9.2

	Has diabetes	Does not have diabetes
Test positive	340 (True positive — TP)	100 (False positive — FP)
Test negative	60 (False negative — FN)	300 (True negative — TN)

a. Sensitivity = TP/(TP+FN) = 340/(340+60) = 85%.   2 marks
b. Specificity = TN/(FP+TN) = 300/(100+300) = 75%.   2 marks
c. Positive Predictive Value = TP/(TP+FP) = 77.2%.   2 marks
d. Negative Predictive Value = TN/(FN+TN) = 83.3%.   2 marks
e. Prevalence = Has Diabetes/Has Diabetes + Does not Have Diabetes =   2 marks
    400/800 = 50%.

26)

a. Cluster headache.   1 marks
b. Any 4 from: 4 marks
    • Onset of headaches >50 years.
    • Thunderclap headache — subarachnoid haemorrhage.
    • Neurological symptoms or signs.
    • Meningism.
    • Immunosuppression or malignancy.
    • Red eye and haloes around lights — acute angle closure glaucoma.
    • Worsening symptoms.
    • Symptoms of temporal arteritis.
    • Worse in the morning or bending forward.
    • Cough-initiated headache.
c. Any 2 from: 2 marks
    • Oxygen.
    • Sumatriptan.
    • Zolmitriptan.
d. Any 1 from: 1 mark
    • Corticosteroids.
    • Verapamil.
    • Lithium.
e. Any 2 from: 2 marks
    • Alcohol.
    • Petrol.

- Paint.
- Perfume.
- Heat.
- Smoking.

27)

a. Ischaemic stroke.   1 mark
b. Right posterior cerebral artery stroke.   1 mark
c. Any 3 from: 3 marks
   - Severe uncontrolled hypertension.
   - Prior ischaemic stroke.
   - Major surgery within 3 weeks ago.
   - Recent internal haemorrhage (within 2 and 4 weeks).
   - Pregnancy.
   - Active peptic ulcer.
   - Current use of anticoagulants.
d. Any 3 from: 3 marks
   - Prior intracranial haemorrhage.
   - Intracranial malformation.
   - Intracranial neoplasm.
   - Ischaemic stroke within 3 months.
   - Suspected dissection.
   - Recent surgery.
   - Recent head trauma.
   - Bleeding diathesis.
e. Any 2 from: 2 marks
   - Clopidogrel (P2Y12 receptor inhibitor).
   - Aspirin.
   - Dipyridamole (phosphodiesterase inhibitors).
   - Warfarin.
   - Direct oral anticoagulants (DOACs), e.g. rivaroxaban.
   - Statins (HMG-CoA reductase inhibitor).

- Calcium channel blockers.
- ACE inhibitors.
- Angiotensin receptor blockers.
- Thiazide diuretics.

28)

a. Gilbert's syndrome.   1 mark
b. 1 mark for each category with two correct examples: 3 marks
   - Pre-hepatic: sickle cell, hereditary spherocytosis, pernicious anaemia, thalassaemia, haemolytic disease of the newborn, G6PD deficiency.
   - Hepatic: viral hepatitis, autoimmune hepatitis, drug-induced hepatitis, alcohol-induced hepatitis, primary biliary cirrhosis, primary sclerosing cholangitis, Gilbert's syndrome, Crigler-Najjar syndrome, right heart failure, acute Budd-Chiari syndrome, Wilson's disease, non-alcoholic fatty liver disease, leptospirosis, Cytomegalovirus, Epstein-Barr virus, hepatocellular carcinoma, decompensated chronic liver disease.
   - Post-hepatic: biliary stricture, biliary atresia, gallstones, pancreatitis, primary sclerosing cholangitis, cholangiocarcinoma, carcinoma of pancreas head.
c. Urine — dark colour.   2 marks
   Stool — normal colour.
d. Bilirubin uridine diphosphate glucuronosyltransferase.   1 mark
e. Any 3 from: 3 marks
   - Kernicterus.
   - Cholangitis.
   - Malabsorption.
   - Hepatic or renal failure.
   - Hepatocellular carcinoma.
   - Cholangiocarcinoma.

29)

a. Any 3 from: 3 marks
- Orthopnoea.
- Paroxysmal nocturnal dyspnoea.
- Palpitations.
- Angina.
- Syncope.
- Chronic cardiac failure.

b. Early diastolic murmur.   2 marks

c. Any 2 from: 2 marks
- Wide pulse pressure
- Corrigan's sign — visible distention and collapse of carotid arteries in the neck.
- De Musset's sign — head bobbing with each heartbeat.
- Duroziez's sign — finger compressing the femoral artery gives a systolic murmur.
- Quincke's sign — pulsations are seen in the nail bed with each heartbeat when the nail bed is lightly compressed.
- Traube's sign — 'pistol shot' sound heard when a stethoscope is placed over the femoral artery during systole and diastole.
- Muller's sign — uvula pulsations are seen with each heartbeat.

d. Any 1 from: 1 mark
- ECG.
- Chest X-ray.
- Echocardiogram.
- Cardiac catheterisation.

e. Any 2 from: 2 marks
- Ascending aortic arch dissection.
- Infective endocarditis.
- Chest trauma.
- Prosthetic aortic valve failure.
- Marfan syndrome.

- Ehlers-Danlos syndrome.
- Ankylosing spondylitis.
- Takayasu arteritis.
- Rheumatoid arthritis.
- Systemic lupus erythematosus.
- Syphilis.
- Infective endocarditis.
- Hypertension.
- Pseudoxanthoma elasticum.
- Osteogenesis imperfecta.

30)

a. Parkinson's disease.   1 mark
b. Any 3 from: 3 marks
- Postural instability.
- Difficulty initiating.
- Micrographia.
- Speech changes.
- Cognitive impairment.
- Depression.
- Hallucinations.
- Brisk reflex.
- Constipation.
- Sleep disorder.
c. Loss of dopaminergic neurons (1 mark) within the substantia nigra (1   2 marks
mark).
d. Any 2 from: 2 marks
- Dopamine agonists.
- Monoamine oxidase-B inhibitors.
- Anticholinergics.
- Catechol-O-methyltransferase inhibitors.

e.   Any 2 from: 2 marks
- On-off fluctuations.
- Dyskinesia.
- Weaning off phenomenon.
- Psychosis.
- Hallucinations.

31)

a.   Inferior ST segment elevation myocardial infarction (STEMI).   1 mark
b.   Right coronary artery.   1 mark
c.   Any 3 from: 3 marks
- Loading with aspirin and one other antiplatelet agent (typically ticagrelor or clopidogrel).
- Nitrates (glyceryl trinitrate sublingual or infusion).
- Diamorphine.
d.   Any 1 from: 1 mark
- Primary percutaneous coronary intervention.
- Thrombolysis.
e.   Any 4 from: 4 marks
- Pericarditis.
- Myocardial rupture.
- Tamponade.
- Mitral regurgitation.
- Septal defects.
- Arrhythmias.
- Ventricular failure.
- Embolism.
- Dressler's syndrome.
- Death.

32)

a.	Asthma.	1 mark
b.	Any 3 from:	3 marks

- House dust mite.
- Pollen.
- Domestic pets.
- Cold air.
- Exercise.
- Emotions.
- Cigarette smoke.
- Infections.
- Drugs such as NSAIDs or β-blockers.

c.	Obstructive pattern (reduced FEV1:FVC ratio).	1 mark
d.	Inhaled short-acting β2-agonists, e.g. salbutamol.	1 mark
e.	Step 2: regular preventer therapy — add inhaled corticosteroids 200-800µg/day.	4 marks

Step 3: initial add-on therapy — add inhaled long-acting β2-agonists, e.g. salmeterol.

Step 4: persistent poor control — increase inhaled corticosteroids up to 2000µg/day or addition of fourth drug, e.g. leukotriene receptor antagonists, slow-release theophylline, β2 agonists.

Step 5: continuous or frequent use of oral steroids — addition of daily steroid tablets at lowest dose possible to maintain adequate control and referral to specialist care.

33)

a.	Lynch syndrome or hereditary non-polyposis colorectal cancer (HNPCC).	1 mark
b.	Any 4 from:	4 marks

- At least three family members must have a cancer associated with hereditary non-polyposis colorectal cancer — colorectal, endometrial, urothelial or small bowel cancer.

- One must be a first degree relative of the other two.
- At least two successive generations must be affected.
- At least one of the relatives with cancers associated with HNPCC must have been diagnosed before the age of 50 years.
- Familial adenomatous polyposis (FAP) should be excluded.

c.   Any 2 from: 2 marks
- Familial adenomatous polyposis (FAP).
- Juvenile polyposis.
- Peutz-Jeghers syndrome.
- MYH-associated polyposis (MAP).
- Cowden syndrome.

d.   Microsatellite instability — MSH2. MLH1, MSH6, PMS2.   1 mark

e.   Any 2 from: 2 marks
- Gastric cancer.
- Endometrial cancer.
- Ovarian cancer.
- Pancreatic cancer.
- Prostate cancer.
- Small bowel cancer.
- Renal cancer.

34)

a.   Fever.   3 marks
     Weight loss >10% in 6 months.
     Night sweats.

b.   Any 2 from: 2 marks
- Enlarged lymph nodes.
- Splenomegaly.
- Hepatomegaly.

c.   Ultrasound-guided biopsy.   1 mark

d.   Any 3 from: 3 marks
- Chest X-ray.
- CT chest.

- CT abdomen.
- CT pelvis.
- Bone marrow biopsy.
e. Ann-Arbor staging.   1 mark

35)

a. Nephritic syndrome.   1 mark
b. Any 5 from: 5 marks
   - Granulomatosis with polyangiitis (Wegener's granulomatosis).
   - Churg-Strauss syndrome.
   - Microscopic polyangiitis.
   - Goodpasture's syndrome.
   - Membranoproliferative glomerulonephritis.
   - IgA nephropathy.
   - Post-infectious glomerulonephritis.
   - Systemic lupus erythematosus.
   - Subacute bacterial endocarditis.
   - Hepatitis C.
   - Shunt nephritis.
   - Henoch-Schönlein purpura.
   - Haemolytic uraemic syndrome.
   - Rapidly progressive glomerulonephritis.
   - Cryoglobulinaemia.
c. Any 2 from: 2 marks
   - Renal biopsy.
   - Blood culture.
   - Antinuclear antibody (ANA).
   - Anti-glomerular basement membrane antibody (anti-GBM).
   - Anti-neutrophil cytoplasmic antibody (ANCA).
   - Serum complement.
d. Any 1 from: 1 mark
   - Metabolic acidosis.
   - Refractory hyperkalaemia.

- Volume overload.
- Altered mental status.
- Seizures.
- Pericarditis.
- Intractable nausea and vomiting.

e. Goodpasture's syndrome. 1 mark

36)

a. Alcohol. 1 mark

b. Any 4 from: 4 marks
- Gallstones.
- Trauma.
- Scorpion stings.
- Steroids.
- Mumps.
- Malignancy.
- Autoimmune.
- Hypercalcaemia.
- Hypertriglycerides.
- ERCP.
- Drugs such as hormone replacement therapy.
- Contraceptive pill.
- Azathioprine.
- Sulfamethoxazole.
- Trimethoprim.

c. Any 1 from: 1 mark
- Amylase.
- Lipase.

d. Any 2 from: 2 marks
- Shock.
- Acute respiratory distress syndrome (ARDS).
- Sepsis.

- Disseminated intravascular coagulation (DIC).
- Renal failure.

e. Any 2 from: 2 marks
   - Pancreatic pseudocyst.
   - Pancreatic necrosis.
   - Abscess.
   - Splenic artery thrombosis.
   - Duodenal artery thrombosis.
   - Chronic pancreatitis.

37)

a. Asymmetry.   5 marks
   Irregular border.
   Colour change.
   Diameter greater than 6mm.
   Evolving lesion.

b. Any 2 from: 2 marks
   - Increasing age.
   - Previous skin cancer.
   - Multiple naevi.
   - Family history.
   - Parkinson's disease.
   - Skin pigmentation (fair skin, freckled complexion, burns easily).

c. Any 1 from: 1 mark
   - Lentigo maligna.
   - Superficial spreading.
   - Nodular.
   - Acral.
   - Lentiginous.

d. BRAF V600 mutation.   1 mark

e.   Any 1 from: 1 mark
   ● Skin excision.
   ● Mohs surgery.
   ● Sentinel lymph node biopsy.

38)

a.   Any 3 from: 3 marks
   ● Multiparity.
   ● Multiple sexual partners.
   ● Early first intercourse.
   ● Immunosuppression.
   ● Smoking.
   ● History of other sexually transmitted infections.
   ● Human papilloma virus infection.
   ● Family history of cervical cancer.
   ● Oral contraceptive pill.

b.   Human papilloma virus (HPV).   1 mark

c.   Any 2 from: 2 marks
   ● 16.
   ● 18.
   ● 31.
   ● 33.
   ● 34.
   ● 35.
   ● 39.
   ● 45.
   ● 51.
   ● 52.
   ● 56.
   ● 58.
   ● 59.
   ● 66.

- 68.
- 70.

d. Any 3 from: 3 marks
  - Attending cervical screening.
  - Use of barrier method contraception.
  - Limiting the number of sexual partners.
  - Smoking cessation.

e. Large loop excision of the transformation zone (LLETZ).   1 mark

39)

a. Any 5 from: 5 marks
  - Fever of ≥5 days' duration.
  - Bilateral non-suppurative conjunctivitis.
  - Erythema.
  - Mucosal involvement — erythema, fissure, crusting.
  - Strawberry tongue.
  - Polymorphous non-vesicular rash.
  - Lymphadenopathy.

b. Any 1 from: 1 mark
  - Cardiac angiogram.
  - Echocardiogram.
  - CT scan.
  - Ultrasound.
  - Electrocardiogram.
  - CRP.
  - ESR.
  - Liver function tests.
  - Full blood count.

c. Any 1 from: 1 mark
  - Scarlet fever.
  - Juvenile rheumatoid arthritis.
  - Paediatric multisystem inflammatory syndrome.

d. Any 2 from: 2 marks
- Aspirin.
- Immunoglobulins.
- Corticosteroids.

e. Any 1 from: 1 mark
- Coronary artery aneurysms.
- Pericarditis.
- Myocarditis.
- Myositis.
- Pancreatitis.
- Otitis media.
- Hepatitis.
- Gallbladder hydrops.
- Mild aortic root dilatation.
- Myocardial infarction.
- Peripheral gangrene.

40)

a. Bacterial meningitis.   2 marks
b. *Neisseria meningitidis*.   1 mark
c. Any 3 from: 3 marks
- Opening pressure >30cm/H_2O.
- Turbid appearance.
- Protein >1g/L (raised).
- Glucose <2.2mmol/L (low).
- White cell count >500 cells/µL — predominantly neutrophils.

d. Any 2 from: 2 marks
- Normal opening pressure.
- Fibrin web appearance.
- Protein 0.1-0.5g/L (normal to high).
- Normal glucose.
- Negative Gram stain.

e. Any 2 from: 2 marks
- Normal opening pressure.
- Clear appearance.
- Protein <1g/L (mildly increased).
- Normal glucose.
- Negative Gram stain.
- White cell count <500 cells/μL — predominantly lymphocytes.

Chapter 10

Abdominal X-ray
ANSWERS

Interpretation answers

The interpretation of the following abdominal X-rays are shown overleaf:

Abdominal X-ray 1
Abdominal X-ray 2
Abdominal X-ray 3
Abdominal X-ray 4
Abdominal X-ray 5

Abdominal X-ray answer 1:

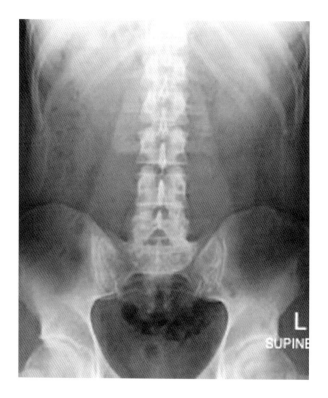

Image quality: AP view; vertebrae visible; no evidence of rotation; costophrenic angles just visible.

Air: no free air visible.

Bowels: normal appearances of small and large bowel.

Calcifications: no calcifications noted.

Densities: normal appearances of abdominal organs.

Everything else: no foreign bodies, lines, contraceptive devices or artefacts present.

Diagnosis: normal abdominal X-ray.

Abdominal X-ray answer 2:

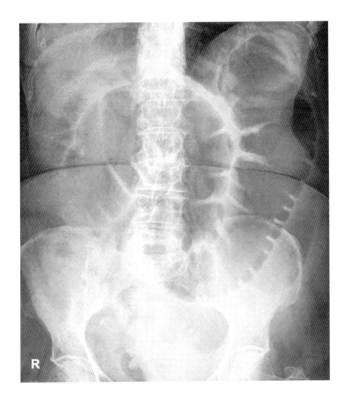

Image quality: AP view; vertebrae visible; no evidence of rotation; costophrenic angles just visible.

Air: no free air visible.

Bowels: dilated loops of bowel; peripheral in nature; bowel >6cm; haustra visible.

Calcifications: no calcifications noted.

Densities: normal appearances of abdominal organs.

Everything else: no foreign bodies, lines, contraceptive devices or artefacts present.

Diagnosis: large bowel obstruction.

Abdominal X-ray answer 3:

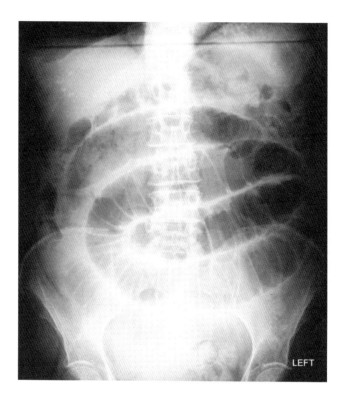

Image quality: AP view; vertebrae visible; no evidence of rotation; costophrenic angles just visible.

Air: no free air visible.

Bowels: dilated loops of bowel; central in nature; bowel >3cm; valvulae conniventes visible.

Calcifications: no calcifications noted.

Densities: normal appearances of abdominal organs.

Everything else: no foreign bodies, lines, contraceptive devices or artefacts present.

Diagnosis: small bowel obstruction.

Abdominal X-ray answer 4:

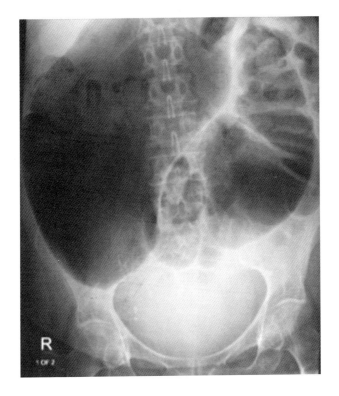

Image quality: AP view; vertebrae visible; no evidence of rotation.

Air: no free air visible.

Bowels: dilated mass in the right upper quadrant arising from the right iliac fossa.

Calcifications: no calcifications noted.

Densities: normal appearances of abdominal organs.

Everything else: no foreign bodies, lines, contraceptive devices or artefacts present.

Diagnosis: sigmoid volvulus.

Abdominal X-ray answer 5:

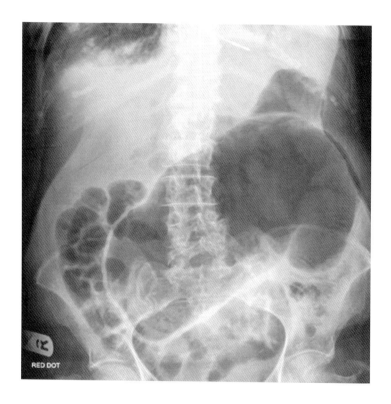

Image quality: AP view; vertebrae visible; no evidence of rotation; costophrenic angle present on right.

Air: no free air visible.

Bowels: dilated mass in the left lower quadrant arising from the left iliac fossa.

Calcifications: no calcifications noted.

Densities: normal appearances of abdominal organs.

Everything else: nasogastric tube present in the stomach.

Diagnosis: caecal volvulus.

Chapter 11

Chest X-ray
ANSWERS

Interpretation answers

The interpretation of the following chest X-rays are shown overleaf:

Chest X-ray 1

Chest X-ray 2

Chest X-ray 3

Chest X-ray 4

Chest X-ray 5

Chest X-ray 6

Chest X-ray 7

Chest X-ray answer 1:

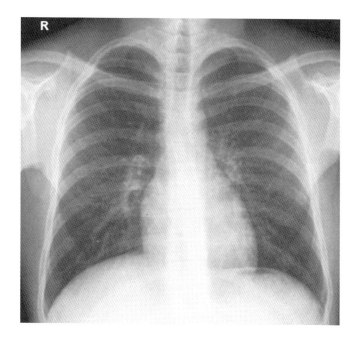

Image quality: not rotated; 6 anterior ribs; PA film; and adequate exposure.
Airway: trachea central; hila symmetrical and bronchi clear; carina visualised; clear costophrenic angles.
Breathing: lung fields clear with no evidence of pleural effusion.
Circulation: cardiothoracic ratio <50%; aortic knuckle and aortopulmonary window clear.
Diaphragm: no free air under the diaphragm.
Everything else: no lines or tubes present; soft tissue and bony surfaces normal.
Diagnosis: normal chest X-ray.

Chest X-ray answer 2:

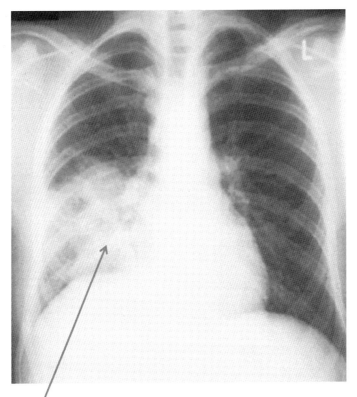

Right-sided consolidation

Image quality: not rotated; 6 anterior ribs; PA film; and adequate exposure.

Airway: trachea central; hila symmetrical and bronchi clear; carina visualised; clear costophrenic angles.

Breathing: right-sided consolidation; left lung field clear.

Circulation: cardiothoracic ratio <50%; aortic knuckle and aortopulmonary window clear.

Diaphragm: no free air under the diaphragm.

Everything else: no lines or tubes present; soft tissue and bony surfaces normal.

Diagnosis: right lower lobe pneumonia.

Chest X-ray answer 3:

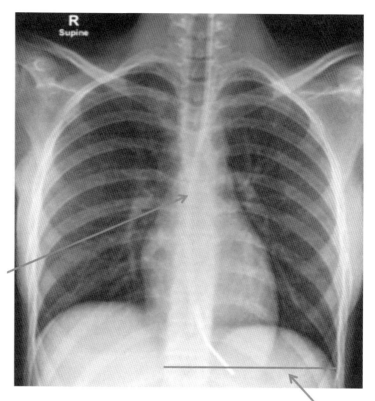

NG tube

Lower border of the diaphragm

Image quality: not rotated; 6 anterior ribs; PA film; and adequate exposure.
Airway: trachea central; hila symmetrical and bronchi clear; carina visualised; clear costophrenic angles.
Breathing: lung fields clear with no evidence of pleural effusion.
Circulation: cardiothoracic ratio <50%; aortic knuckle and aortopulmonary window clear.
Diaphragm: no free air under the diaphragm.
Everything else: tip of the NG tube lying centrally and at a level below the diaphragm.
Diagnosis: correctly positioned NG tube.

Chest X-ray answer 4:

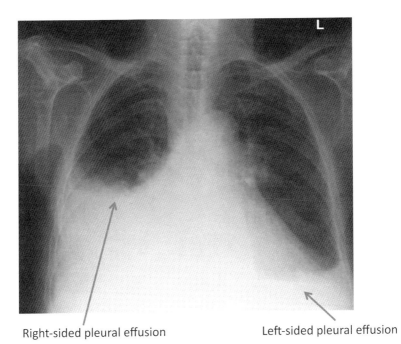

Right-sided pleural effusion   Left-sided pleural effusion

Image quality: not rotated; 5 anterior ribs; PA film; and adequate exposure.

Airway: trachea central; hila symmetrical; carina not visualised; clear costophrenic angles.

Breathing: large right-sided pleural effusion and small left pleural effusion.

Circulation: unable to assess cardiothoracic ratio; aortic knuckle and aortopulmonary window clear.

Diaphragm: unable to assess the diaphragm due to fluid meniscus.

Everything else: no lines or tubes present; soft tissue and bony surfaces normal.

Diagnosis: large right-sided pleural effusion and small left-sided pleural effusion.

Chest X-ray answer 5:

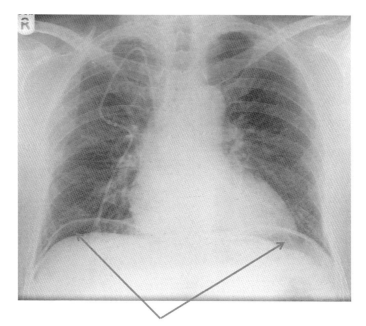

Free air under the diaphragm

Image quality: not rotated; 6 anterior ribs; PA film; and adequate exposure.
Airway: trachea central; hila symmetrical and bronchi clear; carina visualised; clear costophrenic angles.
Breathing: lung fields clear with no evidence of pleural effusion.
Circulation: cardiothoracic ratio <50%; aortic knuckle and aortopulmonary window clear.
Diaphragm: free air under the diaphragm.
Everything else: no lines or tubes present; soft tissue and bony surfaces normal.
Diagnosis: bowel perforation.

Chest X-ray answer 6:

Right-sided pneumothorax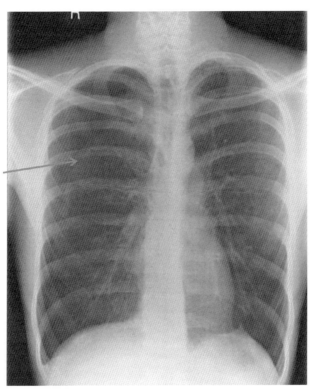

Image quality: not rotated; 8 anterior ribs; PA film; and adequate exposure.
Airway: trachea central; hila symmetrical and bronchi clear; carina visualised; clear costophrenic angles.
Breathing: moderately sized right-sided pneumothorax; left lung field clear.
Circulation: cardiothoracic ratio <50%; aortic knuckle and aortopulmonary window clear.
Diaphragm: free air under the diaphragm.
Everything else: no lines or tubes present; soft tissue and bony surfaces normal.
Diagnosis: right-sided pneumothorax.

Chest X-ray answer 7:

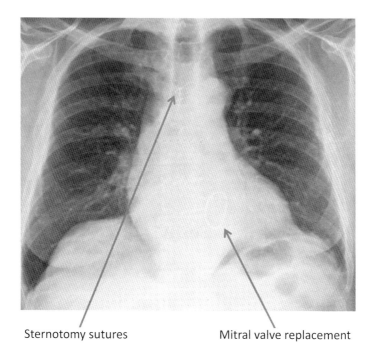

Sternotomy sutures   Mitral valve replacement

Image quality: not rotated; 7 anterior ribs; PA film; and adequate exposure.

Airway: trachea central; hila symmetrical and bronchi clear; carina visualised; clear costophrenic angles.

Breathing: lung fields clear; minor left basal atelectasis.

Circulation: cardiothoracic ratio ~50%; aortic knuckle and aortopulmonary window clear.

Diaphragm: no free air under the diaphragm.

Everything else: mitral valve replacement present; sternotomy sutures present.

Diagnosis: mitral valve replacement.

Chapter 12

ECG
ANSWERS

Interpretation answers

The interpretation of the following ECGs are shown overleaf:

ECG 1
ECG 2
ECG 3
ECG 4
ECG 5
ECG 6
ECG 7
ECG 8
ECG 9
ECG 10

ECQ answer 1:

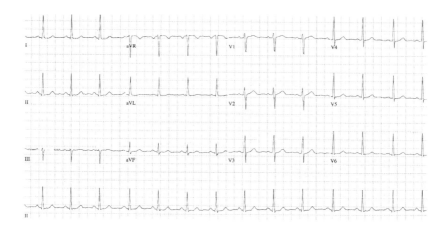

Heart rate: 80 beats per minute.

Rhythm: regular.

Cardiac axis: normal.

P wave morphology: P waves with subsequent QRS; normal duration, direction and shape.

PR interval: 0.16s.

QRS complex morphology: normal width, height and morphology.

ST segment: isoelectric.

T wave morphology: normal.

Overall: normal sinus rhythm.

ECG answer 2:

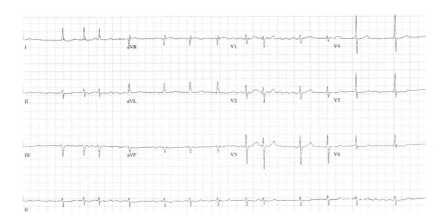

Heart rate: 89 beats per minute.
Rhythm: irregularly irregular.
Cardiac axis: normal.
P wave morphology: absent.
PR interval: N/A.
QRS complex morphology: normal width, height and morphology.
ST segment: isoelectric.
T wave morphology: normal.
Overall: atrial fibrillation.

ECG answer 3:

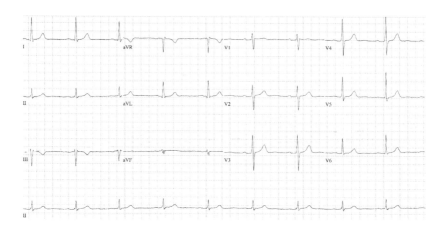

Heart rate: 55 beats per minute.

Rhythm: regular.

Cardiac axis: normal.

P wave morphology: P waves with subsequent QRS; normal duration, direction and shape.

PR interval: 0.2s.

QRS complex morphology: normal width, height and morphology.

ST segment: isoelectric.

T wave morphology: normal.

Overall: sinus bradycardia.

ECG answer 4:

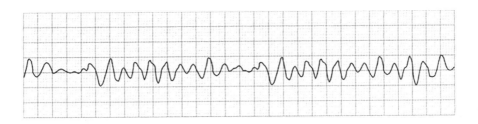

Heart rate: 260 beats per minute — 26 R waves in 6 seconds.

Rhythm: irregular.

Cardiac axis: can't be determined.

P wave morphology: absent.

PR interval: N/A.

QRS complex morphology: can't be determined.

ST segment: can't be determined.

T wave morphology: can't be determined.

Overall: ventricular fibrillation.

ECG answer 5:

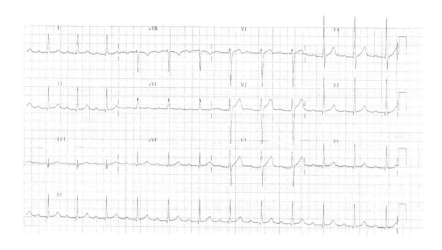

Heart rate: 75 beats per minute.

Rhythm: regular.

Cardiac axis: normal.

P wave morphology: P waves with subsequent QRS; normal duration, direction and shape.

PR interval: 292ms.

QRS complex morphology: normal width, height and morphology.

ST segment: isoelectric.

T wave morphology: normal.

Overall: first degree heart block.

ECG answer 6:

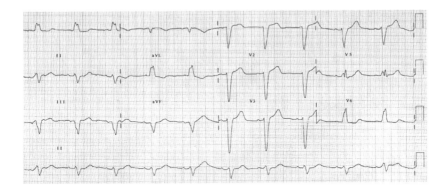

Heart rate: 60 beats per minute.

Rhythm: regular.

Cardiac axis: left axis deviation.

P wave morphology: P waves with subsequent QRS; normal duration, direction and shape.

PR interval: 0.18s.

QRS complex morphology: rS complex in V1; broad 'M'-shaped R wave in V6; QRS >0.12s.

ST segment: ST elevation — appropriate discordance*.

T wave morphology: upright T waves in V1 — appropriate discordance*.

Overall: left bundle branch block.

---

* Appropriate discordance: ST segments and T waves always go in the opposite direction to the QRS direction.

ECQ answer 7:

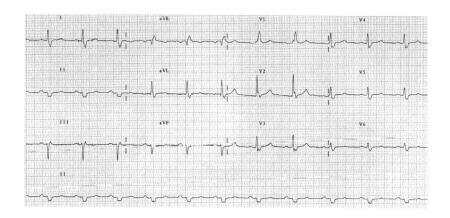

Heart rate: 70 beats per minute.

Rhythm: regular.

Cardiac axis: right axis deviation.

P wave morphology: P waves with subsequent QRS; normal duration, direction and shape.

PR interval: 0.16s.

QRS complex morphology: RSR' pattern V1 (M-shaped QRS); wide S wave in V6; broad QRS >0.12s.

ST segment: ST depression in V1-V3 leads.

T wave morphology: normal.

Overall: right bundle branch block.

ECG answer 8:

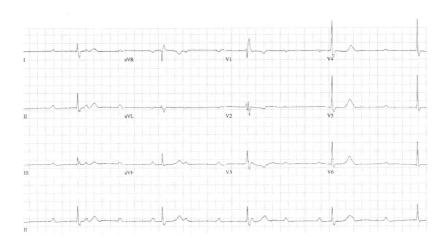

Heart rate: 29 beats per minute.

Rhythm: regular but P and QRS rate are different.

Cardiac axis: normal.

P wave morphology: abnormal; not every P wave is followed by a QRS.

PR interval: unable to assess.

QRS complex morphology: widened QRS complex >0.12s; right bundle branch block.

ST segment: isoelectric.

T wave morphology: normal.

Overall: third degree heart block (complete heart block).

ECG answer 9:

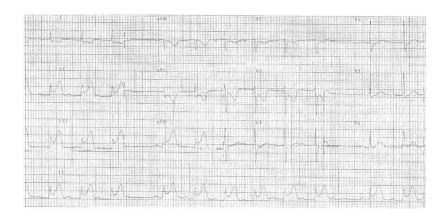

Heart rate: 75 beats per minute.

Rhythm: regular.

Cardiac axis: normal.

P wave morphology: P waves with subsequent QRS; normal duration, direction and shape.

PR interval: 0.2 seconds — seen in lead V2.

QRS complex morphology: normal, but ST segment elevated.

ST segment: ST elevation in leads II, III, aVF with reciprocal ST depression in leads aVL and V1-V6.

T wave morphology: reciprocal T wave inversion in aVL.

Overall: inferior STEMI.

ECG answer 10:

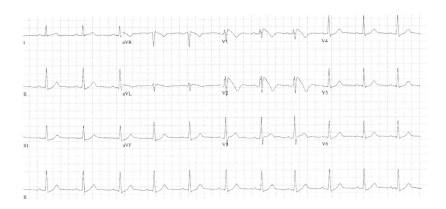

Heart rate: 68 beats per minute.

Rhythm: regular.

Cardiac axis: normal.

P wave morphology: P waves with subsequent QRS; normal duration, direction and shape.

PR interval: 0.17s.

QRS complex morphology: ST elevation in V1-V3 followed by a negative T wave.

ST segment: T elevation in V1-V3 followed by a negative T wave.

T wave morphology: negative T waves in V1-V3.

Overall: Brugada syndrome Type I.